M000188887

Just Motivate Me

— FOR FITNESS —

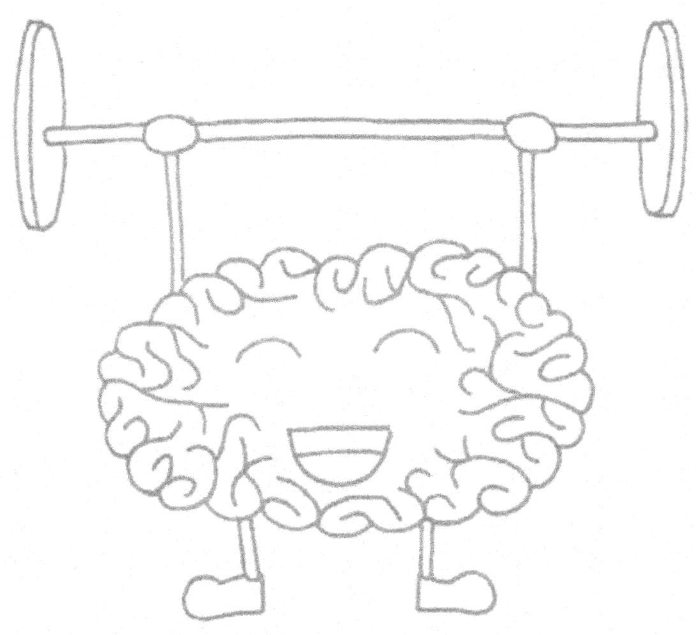

Train your mind to train your body.

RUSSELL COTTER

The content in this book makes no claim to being medically authorized or supported and as with any form of improvement towards fitness, professional medical advice should always be sought.

The information on this book is mostly anecdotal and insights provided are derived from reflection on personal experiences and observations.

For more information, please visit www.justmotivateme.org

ISBN PRINT 978-1-09837-522-5 | ISBN eBOOK 978-1-09837-523-2

Contents

Dedication

I dedicate this book to my daughter, Cassandra, my son, Matthew, and my partner and best friend ever, Seema. All of you are my reasons for trying to be the best that I can be. Now and for the future

I also dedicate this book to you, the readers, especially to those who are frustrated with their low motivation or lack of progress in becoming fit. I have experienced that same frustration, the bouts of guilt and the doubts of my own abilities. It can be very soul sucking and difficult. Finally, I dedicate this to my future self, the "me" in the future who will thank the "me" of today for figuring out how to keep motivated.

Introduction

It can be tough and disheartening to keep restarting, to go through life wanting to improve your fitness, spending money, feeling like you cannot attain your goals and going through periods of guilt that make low motivation even lower.

So now you must be thinking, *Here we go …* another *book on fitness? Give me a break! Why will this one be any different?*

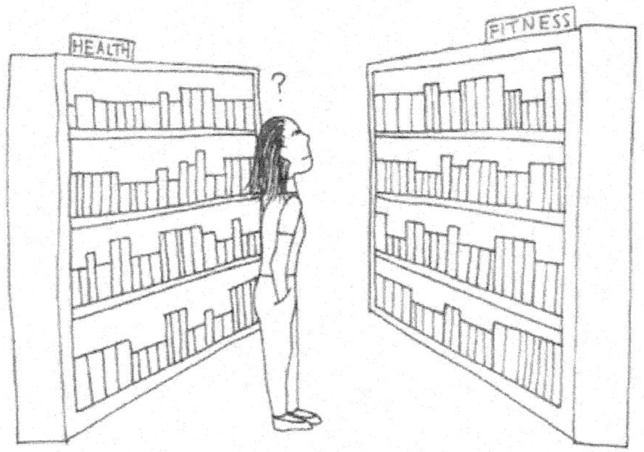

Will I ever find one that works for me?

Several years ago, I turned fifty, and it was an interesting time for me. I clearly remember sixth grade, talking about the year 2000 with my mates and how we would all be thirty-six years of age. To me as a twelve-year-old, this seemed like a distant time, and the idea of being thirty-six gave me pause. How would it feel to be *that* old?

Now, back to the future…

Fast-forward to 2014, and as a fifty-year-old, I did what many fifty-year-olds do and took a little time for reflection. Did I feel old? Did I feel healthy and young, or did I feel like someone who was one stroke away from the nearest old folks' retirement village? It was a moment of reflection, mixed with feelings of slight anxiety, thoughts of promise and opportunity, and curiosity about what my "future self" would or *could* be like.

Where I arrived was a place of assured and confident satisfaction with *where* I was, *who* I was and the life of experiences that trailed behind me. I had traveled around five continents, experienced many lifestyles and occupations, met many people and overcome many life challenges. A few short months into my fiftieth year, I would be doing my final testing for a first-degree black belt in martial arts. Introspection can be a powerful thing because it can lead to reasserting knowledge about your past and present "self" so you can apply it to what you desire your "future self" to be.

I think it was at this point when I considered my own attitudes around personal fitness. I began to realize my obligation to my "future self." I considered the things that were necessary now in order to enjoy a future lifestyle with minimal physical constraints. How could I be a father who would not require a lot of additional elder care from my kids? How would it affect my future self-esteem?

While becoming a more deliberate student of myself, I began writing this book around the theme of developing a fit body through *firstly* focusing on the mind, in ways that did more than the conventional texts on exercise, diet and pure grit. I hope you enjoy this book that shares lessons and insights from my journey. It may not apply to some people, but for some it will be the "book they <u>always</u> wanted".

I intend for this book to be for ordinary people who are *not* fitness superstars, super athletes, special forces combat experts or bodybuilders. My book is meant for people who have varying degrees of disposable income, time and life responsibilities, people who may have had scarce parental attention growing up, people who try very hard and constantly battle disappointment in themselves and just think, *What's the point?*

This book is *not* designed to give you hope. My wish is that this book gives you some of my personal insights along with some tools so that you *create hope within yourself* and from that, you and you alone learn how to train your mind to train your body. For me, this is the book I wish I could have given to my eighteen-year-old self, and although I have a few regrets, I think I did pretty well in my journey of developing a healthy and fit body, even through and in spite of the setbacks I experienced along the way.

The content in this book is mostly anecdotal and based on what I have learned, through the school of hard knocks. So, if you need the books with all the buckets of research and graphs and quotations from various academic studies, then maybe you need to broaden your search.

I wrote this book from the point of view of an everyday person who wants to help everyday people. People with hopes, frustrations, anxieties and complex circumstances that make motivation for exercise difficult to muster.

Now, what about you?

If you are that super athlete, or that seasoned and fit combat veteran, or someone who trains as part of making a living, then this book may be less for you, but, it may more valuable for the people you work with, train with or depend upon.

On the other hand, if you are a regular person putting in eight or more hours a day working a regular job, or a student readying yourself for future life, or even someone who just wants to figure out how they can make themselves more at ease with exercise, then this book is for you.

You are the person who may not be a super driven individual, but you want your body to feel alive with energy. You are the person who *wants* to feel confident in your abilities and happy with a vast strength of self-discipline. You may be the person who bought that teal-and-pink yoga mat, that shiny exercise bike with the fancy computer screen and cup-holder or that very alluring sport center membership with the firm belief that fitness was within your grasp.

After one week, one month or one year, you look around and you see that yoga mat still in its original plastic packaging, you see the exercise bike in the corner of your bedroom with some clothes draped over the frame, and every time you open your wallet or purse you can't help but notice that expired sports center membership card and the hundreds of dollars you donated to the cause of abandoned hopes and dreams.

When it comes to finding out how to get yourself fit, there is a lot of information out there. No, not just a lot—I am talking about an *ocean* of literature. There are also videos and posters in many places and social media sites about how to get fit. Web pages, television infomercials and bookshop shelves will all sell you a fitness solution, no matter that their one commercial is directed at an audience of so many different and diverse people. It is so tempting. You see the sculpted and glistening bodies of hired professionals who advertise the products or services you can purchase for just a few easy payments, at a very special price, but only for a very limited time.

You see, these folks through the use of marketing have already discovered that your mind is up for grabs when it comes to fitness. A few easy payments means that the purchase may not be as cost prohibitive as you imagined. The very special price makes you consider if it would be foolish to ignore the bargain you are being offered. The very limited time induces an amygdala (that primitive part of our brains) response for urgency that creates a personal fear of letting something go.

They're not really Bond villains.

Marketers and advertisers have been doing this for a very long time. They know that when it comes to selling things to get you looking good and feeling great, they just need to begin with appealing to and working with your mind.

Now, to be fair, this is not all part of some evil mind control scheme with an organization of garden-variety Bond villains lurking in the shadows of some subterranean complex. It's just that marketers and businesspeople need to be smart about creating value for their customers, employees, proprietors and shareholders.

I say, if your mind really *is* up for grabs, then why shouldn't *you* be the person who has the most access and control over it? Leaving your mind up for grabs to strangers is something you should definitely question. Once you have full control of your own mind and motivations, you can go out and purchase those products and services that are always being advertised. Chances are, though, that when you do end up buying them, you will actually buy the right things for the right reasons and at the right time.

So, what about me?

I now have a gym that I created in my basement, and it is where I do my regular high-intensity workouts. I can admit to you, though—and it is a little embarrassing—that most of the equipment that I now use daily was purchased and hardly ever used at times over the past twenty years! Now that I have trained my mind, I actually use all of that stuff! So why did I buy it in the first place? For the same reasons as most ordinary people. It looked enticing. Seeing it in the shop gave me a rush and a confidence that shiny new things would transform my body and that these "things" was all that was missing.

I reasoned that without this gear, it was no wonder I looked and felt the way I did. The mind is a highly sophisticated machine that is the ultimate reasoning processor. You will almost always come to some understanding or profound insight that you want to believe. Don't feel bad if you experience this. We are all just human, although some may debate that point when discussing my quirky sense of humor or unconventional wisdom.

Yes, like so many consumers with a highly enthusiastic and energetic optimism for becoming fit, I purchased many different devices and weights that have only relatively recently been put to constant use. If this is starting to sound familiar to you, then I have good news for you: there are stories and insights and things to try all through this book! For fitness, I believe that while books can be very useful, it may be better to begin with a conversation.

Finally, what about your personal physician?

A good place to start is a conversation with your personal physician, someone qualified and trained in human anatomy, knowledgeable in general medical conditions and also familiar with your personal chart. Your doctor is someone you can always talk to, and she, he or they may be able to direct you to some things you may want to try in order to safely set you on a healthy path.

I am lucky to have a great personal physician and he along with my dentist are both trusted and essential to helping me understand how I need to manage my health. They are also very nice human beings.

I also suggest that a conversation about your personal fitness needs should be an *ongoing* conversation with your personal physician. Between visits, you get older, your life circumstances may have changed and your ability to do physical activity may also be changing. While it is helpful for accountability, it also helps your physician understand your abilities and the effect that exercise is having on you. Where exercise is bringing improvements to your health, your physician may be a source of positive reinforcement, and where you may be introducing unnecessary risks, your physician may advise you on things you may need to throttle down and adjust so you don't introduce any injuries or strains.

Your journey starts here—not in a gym, not in a sports center and not in a shopping center. Your journey starts with YOU. Always remember that as with all the things you do or become, the journey begins with you. It will occur on a path that you build for yourself while at the same time you travel along it. Your journey will cover many things that you learn about yourself, challenges that present themselves to you and past accomplishments that you may celebrate and build upon. Your path will intersect with people whom you speak with or train with; it will also intersect with life circumstances over which you have varying degrees of control, and it may not always be easy to follow. There will be chances to stop, to deviate or to abandon your place on the path. These are normal things to expect and when things happen, use your mind to figure a way forward.

Become a student of yourself.

Introspection and motivation will be key to the fitness path you build for yourself and the journey you take along it. The public face of motivation is often seen in all of the sources of information that we process, like mass media marketing campaigns, Social Media, television, radio, billboards and junk mail. Motivation mechanics have, to a large degree, been reduced to soundbites to promote a fitness "attitude." "Just do it." "No pain, no gain." "Your body is your temple." These are just some of the better-known examples, but they do little to address the inevitable reality for the mainstream person, which is this: "Exercise is hard, it can be tedious, it can certainly become boring, and at times it is plain exhausting."

Motivation, that is to say, *true* motivation, is a foundational basis for your fitness journey that is often skipped or underserved, and I believe lack of motivation stands in the way of achieving lasting fitness goals. Motivation is the difference between *intending* to be fit and *being* fit. The reason for me writing this book is because I wanted to shine a light on the singular most important aspect of fitness training that has most positively affected my own journey, and that aspect is motivation that you create for yourself through self-understanding.

Motivation and training the mind will get you to acknowledge yourself as the "real deal" when it comes to training your body. I find it important to acknowledge our lack of motivation and our struggles to become motivated because we are not all strong or capable in the things we wish to be. We are not all young, and we are certainly not all willing to do things that we just do not want to do. Effort is something we may tend to avoid, and effort that is exercise, can be even harder for us to *want* to do because it produces no immediate and tangible gratification, especially early in the journey. I realize there are other narratives out there on motivation, even those that pertain to fitness, but I choose to separate my ideas from them because my story is personal and stands on its own.

This book provides a call to action at the end of many chapters. Think of these passages as a way to encourage a little self-accountability for being open-minded and active in your journey. Don't worry—these calls to action are not telling you to get down and do twenty pushups or to run around the block. These calls to action are about introspection, reflection and studying yourself to the point that you develop an awareness of things that help you to get motivated. Where there are calls to be introspective, write down what you discover about yourself in your personal motivation journal. When you find something out about yourself, my advice is "Just write it down."

The deliberate act of writing things down can help you to become more thoughtful in your self-discovery, and once written, those very same journal entries can be used to inspire you to action when it comes to knowing the most effective methods and circumstances that will help your mind to train your body.

Once you have begun to learn more about yourself, to discover your personal motivations and preferences, then those future fitness dollars will be better spent, when you *do* decide to pick up and use that gym membership, or when you hire that personal trainer or buy that very nice yoga mat!

How is this book organized?

This book consists of twenty-two main chapters and five bonus chapters.

The main chapters convey some experiences and insights with a call to action at the end of each. I encourage you to try out the guided journaling in the call-to-action sections at the end of each chapter. Although there is sequence to some chapters, many can be read in the order of your choosing. Find something that sparks your interest.

The bonus chapters are additional thoughts, insights and ideas I feel may also be useful to you to read and consider. In addition to this book, there is a website you may visit and subscribe to at www.justmotivateme.org, and I encourage you to check it out. From time to time, I will post information on events, new videos, tools or ideas, or even just provide forums for the exchange of ideas. The website is constantly evolving as my website skills are growing!

...Oh yeah, and blogs. We will be blogging our hearts out.

"A scout smiles and whistles under all circumstances."

Lord Baden-Powell (1857–1941),
FOUNDER OF THE MODERN SCOUTING MOVEMENT

1

WHAT MOTIVATES ME?

When I was ten years old, I joined the Scout Association of Australia. After a few meetings, and with my first backpack, I went on my very first scout camping trip. I was a kid who enjoyed challenges and sought adventure. I was very excited about the prospect of sleeping out in the open wilderness in tents, having campfires and cooking food, hiking and all of that cool scouting stuff. On my first camping trip, we arrived at our campsite in very low light that was quickly turning into night. The whole campsite was being beaten down by driving rain.

At first, I was okay and told myself that in just five minutes, we would have our tent up, we would be inside and dry, and after the rain eased, maybe we would sit around a campfire. It turned out that none of us had ever set up a tent before, and it was cold. Cold, wet and now, pretty dark. It felt brutal splashing around in the mud trying to set out the tent base, holding flashlights while putting up poles, attaching and securing the guy ropes and then putting up the fly. After about forty minutes of misery, we were just too wet and tired to do anything fun and had no chance of even starting a campfire under the relentless rain. All we could think about was getting into our tents and drying out and then going to sleep.

I remember having two thoughts at the time: *What did I get myself into?* and *If this is as bad an experience as I can ever expect, then I can do more of this scouting thing.* My momentary examination of the current circumstances and the thought of future, more positive outcomes motivated me to stay in scouting for several years. Taking that moment to pause, take stock of the situation and consider my feelings and attitudes was one of the first times in my life that I trained my mind. At no time had I ever considered the profound impact this experience would have on me in future years, but I am glad that being a little introspective from an earlier age has probably benefited me in ways that still surprise me.

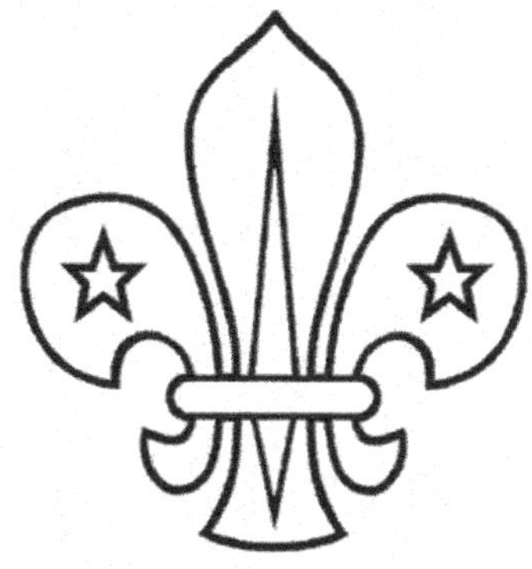

As I have already stated, this book reflects on things I have learned from my journey. Now, that being said, what works for me may not work for the next person. Each person is different, and I strongly feel that if a person is looking for that thing that resonates with them, they should follow that desire. Now, the more viewpoints they open themselves up to, the more likely they will find something they can work with. My viewpoint is unique to me, but you may consider many others. I am just a regular person, not a sculpted muscle man, not someone who indulged in school sports and certainly not a fitness superstar. Viewpoints may be found from a variety of people and include things from their own experiences whether these people are your friends, relatives or acquaintances.

So why do I do the "fitness" thing? Is it because I want to be on the cover of *Sports Illustrated*? No, most definitely not. I do not consider myself a "fitness fanatic," but I do consider myself to have an above average level of fitness for someone of my age and gender. I am by no means a super fit powerhouse, but I am suitably fit to meet the demands of my current lifestyle and the expectations I have for my future self. Yes, that's right, my *future* self. I look at my life with the notion that there is a future version of myself who may be very "judgy" about my present self. He is the version of myself who, if unhappy with his fitness situation, will look back on his life and hold his former self to account for being so slack. Yes, he can be a piece of work! I owe it to my future self to put in the hard yards during *this* time, the time of *now*, to make sure that my future self has a better and more healthy life, even if he is much older and the jokes are still as corny as they are now.

Not everyone thinks about their future self, and there is nothing wrong or unusual about that. The things that most immediately resonate with people are their expectations for their present self-image and overall health. Self-image is definitely a "thing", and most people like to look good or at least presentable. It's just in our nature, but of course there are also many who are not as concerned about their appearance and more concerned with their inner beauty. We are all humans with reasons to be physically and mentally healthy.

For me, I cannot deny my attention to self-image, but I have other reasons that for me are as, if not more important. I want to feel like I can depend on my body to support the activities I want to do and the experiences I wish to have. I have seen friends and relatives who, like me, have very active minds but have bodies that cripple them and crowd their minds with frustrations and regrets that become barriers to their mental happiness. We all get old and the body expires at the end, but wouldn't it be great if we could have a strong body and mind as long as comfortably possible?

I also look at the world around me and see future possibilities for myself. As I age, I cannot deny that certain aspects of physiology degrade with time, but I can definitely help my future self to lessen the effects of aging by making my body strong enough to do the things my mind desires. I also look at my own motivation as something that helps me to help my future loved ones. In the future, my partner will also still want to be dancing to Depeche Mode, and I do not want to be the one sitting still.

I also need to ensure that I do not become burdensome to my kids, whose lives will be filled with activities and possibly, the responsibility of their own families. I know that they will always help me if I need it, but I also feel that I have a responsibility today, to lessen my dependency on them in the future. As parents, I believe that we should always try to help our children as much as we can while also teaching them to help themselves.

So why do I do it? I do it to look good for myself, to feel good in my world, to do good for my loved ones and my community, to be good at things I *want* to do. I also want to avoid my future self kicking my own saggy behind for letting my body down. My future self is likely to be critical of my past self if I don't watch out! That's it. I see and remember the effects that exercise has on me. I use that memory to keep me going. Lastly, my intent is that my future self will have a butt that is firm and pert. It's a non-negotiable for me.

CALL TO ACTION

What motivates you?

Reflect on times and circumstances when you were willing to try out new things, or to try things that seemed hard. It is important to try and understand the aspects of yourself, your life and your circumstances that affect your ability to feel motivated to participate in activities that contribute to fitness.

At the end of this book is a bonus chapter where you can take a personal motivation assessment. It will help you discover your most basic preferences about the settings and factors that make it easier to want to go and do something physical for your health.

In your personal motivation journal, write down the items that you learn on your journey as you begin to adopt calls to action in this book. The act of writing it down will help you to reinforce it in your thinking and provide a record that you may reference for ideas and inspiration in the future.

"Go to any fitness or sporting goods store and see if you can spot the motivation machine. If you cannot find it, go home and look at a mirror instead."

Russell Cotter

2

MOTIVATION IS MENTAL

I remember when I first emigrated to the United States from Australia. Cable television was a new wonder for me to experience, and amongst the extensive variety of shows, there was a home shopping channel. People would present products and for a limited time only you could have the privilege of buying the wonder product of your dreams, by dialing a telephone number, signing up for four easy payments and getting a free set of steak knives to boot. I was entranced by a curved device that you rocked with, back and forth on the floor, to sculpt your body into "washboard abs." It looked simple, the models were not even breaking a sweat and they each had a physique that was being associated with the use of this new wonder-machine.

At the time, my abs were more like "washing *machine* abs," so I purchased one, and after the initial three days of excitement, it was retired to another room with my most sincere belief that I would try it again soon, if *only* I had the time. The idea of the device was exciting, but the excitement was short-lived, along with my motivation.

How many of you reading this now are thinking, *Yep, been there, done that*?

Now, how many times have you seen a commercial for a gym with lean, sweaty bodies pumping up their muscles, or sporting equipment in stores that makes you think, *If I just bought this stability ball and these hand weights, I could get myself in shape*? It is very easy to be sucked into a false sense of motivation by great marketing or enticing products, but once you have signed up for that abs workout video or bought that kettlebell, you soon begin to realize that the rest of it is all on you.

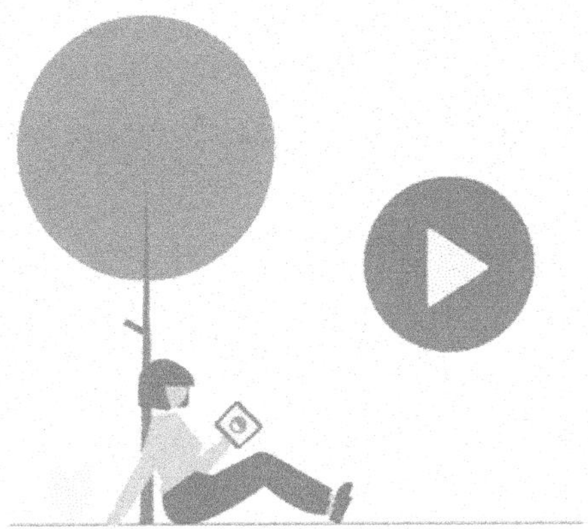

So, it's all up to me?

The commercial you saw for that abs workout video weeks ago, no longer inspires you the way you thought it did, and it certainly doesn't help you want to keep watching the same video over again to put your body through rigorous, repetitive and sometimes painful anguish. Excuses begin to take over and soon, the notion of working out in your living room wearing your shiny spandex is fighting against other thoughts like "I don't have time to workout this morning", "the dog chewed up my workout shoes", I need to get to work earlier today to get ready for that meeting" and all of these excuses can be very strong and valid but, in the end, they become acceptable barriers to avoiding the goal you set out to accomplish.

So, what do you do? You may end up arguing with yourself all over again which can lead to more excuses that are arguably less valid, all the while becoming more frustrated in your head. Accepting excuses and not exploring alternatives can lead you down a very common but slippery slope of detraction from your exercise intentions. More on this to come.

In fact, in my discussions with many friends, they often tell me that the only reason they even keep going to the gym is because they spent all that money on that membership! So, what they are *really* saying is that going to the gym now becomes their punishment and it should serve them right for spending all of that money in the first place—a very negative motivation if ever I heard one.

Some may argue that using an expensive investment to drive self-accountability actually works for them and for their personality and personal preferences it may be a great solution. For others it may lead to guilt. My message to you is this. Learn as much about yourself as you can. You don't need to assume the lotus position and hold your fingers and thumbs together to do this. Find a quiet and peaceful setting to be just by yourself. You may have to ask your spouse to stay and look after the kids for an hour while you find a place. Somewhere away from the responsibilities and distractions of everyday life. You may decide to go for a walk somewhere and ask yourself questions about the things that make you want to pursue fitness as well as the types of things that are barriers or make you procrastinate.

On the surface, and if you are truly being honest, you may determine that you just feel lazy. But could you be saying this because you simply do not have the energy to do more? Being honest is one thing, but try not to be too harsh on yourself either. Telling yourself that you might just feel lazy, is one thing, but asking yourself *why* you feel lazy, may lead you to reveal the deeper understanding you need to get to.

Bruce Lee, the famous martial artist, philosopher and actor, always believed that personal introspection was key in developing the best version of one's self. He never gave a recipe that said that by doing a certain set of exercises or using some new machine, you would improve. His philosophy was that you had to learn about yourself first, to test and determine why you wanted to do certain things and to discover what made them the best choices for your own soul and personality. He was in every way, the person who embodied the warrior spirit, and this has come to be identified in someone so deeply in tune with themselves, that they could face any challenge.

For myself, I also find that I am blessed with a kind of "warrior spirit." I would never compare myself to someone like Bruce Lee, but I do identify with many of his philosophies and ideas. My own spirit of determination is hard to put into words, but I guess my personality has always had a combative aspect to it—not in a mean-spirited sense, but more in the way that I feel I need to challenge myself all the time. I strive to overcome things that seem too hard, especially physical challenges and I accept that work and self-discipline is required. I challenge myself mentally all the time, so it seems that I need the same balance on my physical side for reasons I cannot explain. It's a kind of yin/yang thing with me, and it may explain why I have enjoyed the rigorous challenges that some of my travel exploits, military experience and martial arts training have allowed me to pursue. Everyone is so different, and should endeavor to find out their own personal drivers and barriers, to self-motivation.

You may naturally be self-disciplined, however, if you are not, you may need to develop self-discipline as a tool for yourself. Small habits and routines can be helpful to developing the skills to go a little further, and to be less captive to trivial excuses. It is the fitness of your *mind* that can help your body to overcome things that may seem insurmountable, and it is usually not as easy for many people. You cannot *buy* self-discipline; it is something that you need to create for yourself and then benefit from it, as it grows. When it comes to fitness tenacity, the opposite of self-discipline is weak excuses. Now, that may sound a bit harsh if you consider that in life, we encounter very *valid* reasons to avoid or not pursue physical fitness. You just have to be totally honest with yourself because *you* are the person who can make (and accept) the best excuses you can come up with. If there is one essential message in this book you need to take away, it is this. If you want to develop yourself to be physically fit, you first need to train your mind in order to properly and continuously train your body. Experiment a little, try new things out based on the things you learn about yourself.

CALL TO ACTION

When do you engage in introspection, really looking into yourself and considering who you are and why you do the things you do?

Do you do introspection during the commute to work? Do you do it right after you've managed to put the children down for a nap? Do you do it as you take a long, warm shower? Do you do it at all?

Many of us tend to use our "alone time" to think about everything that concerns our life *around* ourselves but rarely *about* ourselves.

Find the time and place where you can do this. If you have young kids, it may be during your commute to the office or somewhere you can sit down after the kids are in bed.

To train your mind, you have to *sincerely* seek to understand it. A good habit to get into is to write up the things that seem like profound insights or reflections in your personal motivation journal.

“The successful warrior is the average man,
with laser-like focus.”

Bruce Lee

3

MOTIVATION IS PERSONAL

When I left home at the end of my first year in the workforce, I traveled across Australia to take up a new employment opportunity. I was put up in a temporary hostel not far from the center of the city, and it was an exciting part of my life. I experienced no homesickness, just fierce independence and an appetite to learn and try out new things and to burn off energy. I had never done any form of distance running in my youth, having not been very active in sports except for doing the required school physical education programs. The effect of seeing people running on sidewalks outside my building surprised me. I found it *inspiring*. I could not explain *why* it was inspiring, maybe it was the display of energy—something I had an abundance of—or just the way they looked. They also seemed so strong and capable. I think this was something that I must have been wanting to feel more of, at least at a subconscious level.

One day, I decided to put on a pair of sneakers and go for a run. My first self-driven run. Ok, it was a jog. It brought a mix of feelings for me. It was at first fun to feel like I was doing something energetic, enjoying the outdoors and propelling my body under my own will. It did get a little tiring, which didn't surprise me, and at times I slowed down and picked up the pace later when my energy returned. What I learned about myself was that it was good to try new things, to think about the experience and to consider how it felt. I learned that it was also okay to allow myself to adjust my pace, just as long as I was continuously moving. I also realized that I felt even more energized after I returned to the hostel, and soon it became a semi-regular part of my routine in a city where I had few close friends and plenty of time on my hands.

A personal motivation is something to discover without help or prescribed influence from others. Use your own observations, try out a theory and see how it feels. One person's reasons and motivations for working out are seldom the same as the next person. In my journey, motivation has always been deeply personal. This is why, when I see the many books out there that may guarantee results to get your body in shape with some set of exercises or a "method" that involves the latest piece of exercise equipment, or the new set of *rules*, it makes me scratch my head. Mostly I *shake* my head in disbelief. Why? Because everyone is *so* different.

CALL TO ACTION

Do you have desires in your life about who you want to be, what things you want to be capable of? Even ordinary things like having energy to lift yourself out of your couch? Or are you just tired of *being* around things but never or hardly actually *doing* anything?

For the desires you have for yourself, consider carefully what those things are and what they mean to you. Then think about the things you feel are out of reach or possibly unachievable due to your level of fitness. Seek to understand where you struggle to achieve the required level of fitness, and where it seems that *motivation* is holding you back.

Now, write a few things down. Try to align some of your desires with the corresponding physical fitness limitations you have. Write these down as items in your personal motivation journal.

Here are some examples:

My desire is to play golf, but I hold back because the walking may tire me out or swinging golf clubs may not be something my shoulders will endure for an afternoon.

My desire is to avoid being perceived as unable to do activities with my kids or grandkids because I only have short spurts of energy and it limits the amount of *quality* time, I get to spend with them.

"Who dares wins."

Regimental motto of the Special Air Service Regiment (SASR)

4

BEGIN WITH YOUR MIND IN MIND

From my personal experience, I have found that it is extremely important to train your mind in order to train your body.

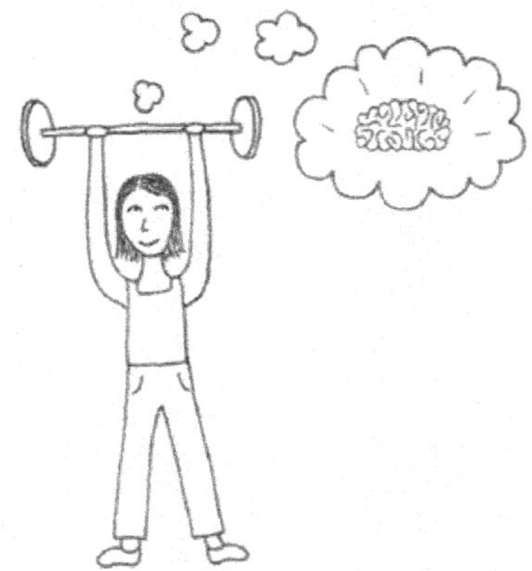

Gotta train my mind to train my body!

I believe that this is the essential first step in overcoming your biggest barrier—your true self. I remember seeing a television documentary on an army selection course many years ago for the Australian Special Forces, and I watched it before I began my own training prior to joining the

Australian Army Reserve. Now, I wasn't joining the special forces, not by a long shot, but I was still taking my role as a combat-ready soldier very seriously, even if my role was in the field of army signals to provide and support brigade communications.

The thing I remember most about that documentary is this. Each soldier was broken down to the very essence of what kept him going mentally. The things that would keep these soldiers going and remain with them, were the things that would matter in life-or-death situations. What I took away from watching that documentary was seeing the difference in soldiers who made it and those who didn't. In the end, it was more to do with brain and less to do with brawn.

The persona that we project to the outside world is usually a mix of myth, truth and ego. It is time to humbly and simply consider the person you are and all of the attributes of your character that affect your willingness to succeed. Humility should not be confused with weakness. In fact, I believe that humility is a healthy and necessary part of the journey to self-actualization and forming a true notion of who you are, what *you* stand for and what *you* are prepared to do to follow through. What you discover about yourself may be a validation but also a surprise; you may find things that help you to understand qualities you didn't know you had or things you regarded about yourself that were exaggerated or inflated. When considering your fitness journey, you need to consider the possibility of what to start with, when to start and most importantly, *why* you are starting at all? What if you encounter a setback? How will that affect you? What will you choose to do and how will you allow it to make you feel?

Whatever you learn about yourself, it will be helpful. It is up to you to *apply* it in the most constructive and realistic way that makes sense and is positive for yourself while considering those around you. Sometimes, it may take less introspection to discover your motivation. For instance, some of us have had a "wake-up call" that makes us reconsider our outlook and attitudes toward the way we think about a healthier lifestyle. For one of my cousins, it was heart related, and after requiring bypass surgery, he decided to quit smoking. My very own and most recent wake-up call was debilitating back pain brought on by nothing in particular other than a deteriorating and unsustained core. Some people may wrestle with the wake-up call but also give in to it and regard it as just another step toward old age. Others may want to fight it and figure out how to address it. Warrior spirit. Definitely a thing – at least for me.

Now, here's something to consider: I believe motivation is *so* personal that what is motivating for one person may not necessarily work for another person. For example, while one person is motivated to exercise in a gym because the energy of others engaged in physical activity stimulates them to action, the gym may be less motivating to a person who is more introverted or uncomfortable about exercising around other people. People with social anxiety disorder may be completely turned off by the notion of being somewhere surrounded by lots of people. Sweaty people at that! The takeaway from this is that when you talk to your friends, relatives or coworkers about the things that "work" for them, keep in mind that those things may not necessarily work for *your* personality, *your* life circumstances, or *your* own lifestyle. In time, as you become an eternal student of yourself, you will learn and master the things that are your triggers to action, and stimulators to commitment. You will also discover the way you will look at and manage through *setbacks* in your journey. Such a crucial and essential part to continuous fitness. Yes, you should always accept and anticipate the reality of setbacks and have some self-understanding that helps you when setbacks present themselves. They are never easy and they always come at times that are most inconvenient and frustrating, but they happen.

CALL TO ACTION

Think about a time in your life when you were motivated to do something because you wanted to become, have, or just accomplish for yourself.

What thoughts or feelings encouraged you to drive forward? What anxieties or pressures made you break through your normal limits? They may be useful to your future self as you tackle fitness motivational challenges and will serve as reminders of motivational challenges that you overcame.

What are some ideas you have about setbacks? What might you feel? What might you be prepared to accept and move forward from?

Make a note of these things in your personal motivation journal.

"Don't stop thinking about tomorrow. Don't stop, it'll soon be here."

Christine McVie, Fleetwood Mac

5

AFFIRMATIONS FOR MOTIVATION

A motivational technique that is fairly popular for some people is the use of affirmations. As you discover the values that resonate most deeply with your core beliefs and inner happiness, you just need to find some simple words or phrases that you feel inspired about. Affirmations are not a magic spell that grants you instant motivation, but they do help you to cultivate a positive attitude that embraces things that have special meaning for you. In fact, neuroscience is revealing that there is physiological proof that just as areas of the brain responsible for movement can be activated, say by the clenching of a fist, the same areas can also be activated with an idle fist and merely *thinking* about it.

When it comes to affirmations, I am reminded of a movie my kids must have watched a zillion times, called *Finding Nemo* by Disney Pixar. It was such a fun film for my kids and for me, with its incredibly funny storyline and characters. It held a special connection for us due to its inclusion of Australian places that are familiar to us. One character, Dory, was a female fish who seemed to have very short-term memory. The one thing she did most notably remember and apply to her journey was a single affirmation:

"Just keep swimming, just keep swimming." I love this example because it is very much like one of my own mental affirmations when it comes to fitness, only for me, especially as I get older, it is more like "Just keep *moving*, just keep *moving*."

Sometimes affirmations may be written as motivational phrases that you place in areas that grab your attention and that serve as a communicative reminder of the things that matter to you most. Try not to use negative words and phrases and see if you can work on the positive. Phrases like "no pain, no gain" may create anxiety over anticipating pain that will only serve to create excuses to *not* participate in physical activity.

When I train, I try to use affirmations of a challenge like "just two extra reps" or "try for one extra minute" that help me prove to myself that I can always do more than I believed I could. When I conquer these challenges, I always get a boost in my feelings of confidence and accomplishment.

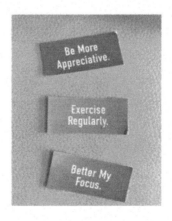

Affirmations for a better you.

Remember, the main theme of this book is training your mind to train your body. Affirmations can have varying degrees of success depending on the individual. Some may feel affirmations work well, some may feel they don't help that much, but like all techniques, reciting affirmations is a great one to keep in your motivational tool kit.

Words of affirmation are something that a lot of people crave to hear from others, especially their spouses, parents, work managers or teachers. As much as hearing affirmations from other people helps, we should never ignore trying to use affirmations on ourselves and to learn more about ourselves by reflecting on how these words affect us.

At the end of the day, I need to reinforce that affirmations are just one technique and this technique alone—in fact, any technique that stands alone—may not be all that you need to get yourself moving. See techniques as tools in your motivational tool kit that you can introduce, use and change out at will as you begin to learn what works and what doesn't and under what set of circumstances.

CALL TO ACTION

What are *your* personal affirmations? Do you ever catch yourself saying or maybe just *thinking* short statements or words just to get you by sometimes? Words that may give you courage, hope or energy to go that little bit further?

Consider the positive things you replay in your mind that may be clues to words that may serve as affirmations. Try to work with this on your own and see if you can come up with two or three words that make good slips to put in your wallet or an inspirational wallpaper for your smartphone. Try and make them positive and not threatening or negative. Think about words or phrases you have heard from others that have been uplifting. These may also be useful to you.

Affirmations can be scripted in forms that are useful in terms of how you will notice them when you need them. You can place them, as I have done, on little cards in your wallet. You might make them into a meme and use it as the wallpaper on your smartphone or computer screen. Sometimes a sticky note on the front door or in the car can also help.

You may just keep one affirmation for fitness that is easy to remember and replay it every time you get up in the morning, like "just keep moving!"

As with all the things you begin to develop as part of training your mind, write these things down in your personal motivation journal. Over time, your journal will become your very own playbook, reference guide and motivation manual.

"The best form of welfare for the troops is first-rate training."

Erwin Rommel

6

PREPARE YOUR MIND

Preparing yourself for any journey is an important step to ensure you meet your objectives. A fitness journey is no exception, and the preparation really should begin with preparing yourself mentally. In 1987, after several years of careful consideration, I decided to join the Australian Army Reserve.

I had many reasons for joining the army, among them, a belief that I had a civic duty to be ready to defend my country against hostile acts, the opportunity to learn new skills and to develop a higher level of fitness for myself, that could only benefit me in mind and body.

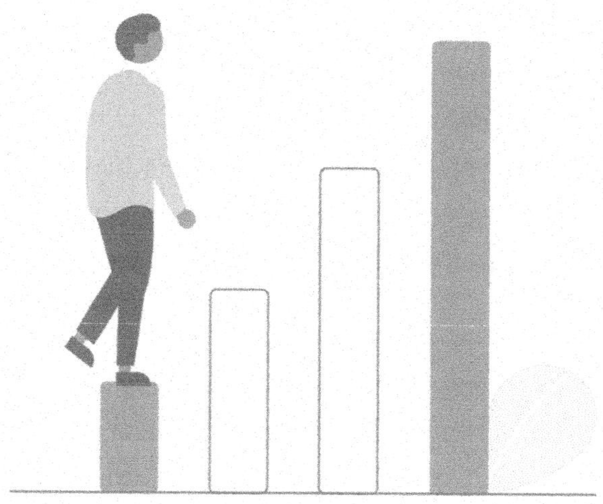

Always upward. Mind and body.

Let's get physical.

My expectations of the upcoming physical aspects for military duty were mostly theoretical and based mostly on documentaries, books and movies. It was this physical aspect that I would say brought about some trepidation as well as the type of excitement that a challenge may bring. When anyone decides to join the Australian Army Reserve, they must first go through administrative processes in order to assess their suitability for the military. Once you have been interviewed, weighed, measured and checked out mentally and physically, if you are accepted, you will receive a letter. The letter conveys congratulations on becoming a recruit in the Australian Army Reserve and explains that you are required to attend basic training (then called the recruit course) at the venue and on the date specified.

Additionally, the letter provides a list of very specific fitness requirements you need to be capable of on entry to the training battalion. The requirements include a table that lists age ranges alongside different exercise expectations for running distance in a certain time, sit-ups, chin-ups, etc. My recruit course was designated 1/88 (pronounced as one of eighty-eight—the first recruit course of the year 1988). These requirements had to be met in early February, about two months after receiving the letter at the beginning of December 1987. As a recruit in early December, I worked with the list of requirements sent to me and created a plan to not only meet the expectations for the Australian army but to also exceed them as a personal challenge to myself. Being an overachiever is something that is a personal trait and something I believe comes from my desire to make things easier on myself in the future, whether that future is weeks, months or years away.

This story is one of my favorite experiences of my life, and now you get to share it with me! Lucky you. So, what did I have to work with? Well, I had my letter of course. I also had my basic army clothes and equipment like belts, webbing harness, water bottles, eating and cooking equipment and shelter for the battlefield. I also had a knee that had been slightly unstable on and off, even after having fairly invasive surgery three years prior. During December, I decided to take my entire four weeks of vacation as a holiday to see my family in Western Australia, and in addition to regular items like clothes and Christmas presents, I took my army duffle bag that contained my webbing and equipment. My personal mission was to meet or exceed the Army Reserve recruit course physical preparation requirements within those four weeks. Stay tuned, more to come on this story …

Preparing your mind is key in establishing and maintaining a personal fitness rhythm. I have learned things about myself that help with my preparation. For example, when I used to jog in the early mornings to keep fit or in the evenings to train for military or social running events, I knew that it helped to have my running gear in a place that was visible to serve as a subtle reminder that I had made a commitment to exercise. I also learned that to prepare myself mentally for running, I just needed to be dressed for it and simply walk out the door. Once I heard the lock in the door click, it was like a trigger to put me in the mode. I never once had a thought to turn around, unlock the door and forget about the whole thing.

This may not work for everyone, but I stress that you need to discover your own personal triggers. I also found out that making an entry in my work calendar served not just as a reminder to leave work on time, but that throughout the week that I was *committed* to training. This definitely helped me prepare for my training in martial arts. I learned something else, similar to the running. Once I stepped over the threshold into the martial arts school, I was able to stop thinking about everything else going on in my life and commit to the next hour ahead of me for stretching, physical training, learning martial arts and practicing with the rest of the class. In summary, many things can help us to prepare. Preparation of our mind helps us to focus, to commit to the activity and to build understanding about the things that we can remind ourselves of that help us stay motivated.

CALL TO ACTION

Think of a time when you were successful in initiating and seeing through a lengthy objective, when your personal planning made a difference, especially in terms of how it affected your mindset to complete the necessary steps and keep on track, and how it made you feel at the end.

You may have had feelings of relief or personal achievement or even a newfound energy to try bigger challenges.

Now, think of a different time when the lack of planning for a lengthy objective made it *unsuccessful* or fraught with frustrations. It might have been a home remodeling experience, or an overseas trip that went terribly wrong, or a wedding that was months in view on the calendar and ended up in some costly or even embarrassing outcomes. What was your motivation for planning things out in your own mind and what lessons—good practices or things to avoid—did you learn?

How will you try to really focus and to concentrate on your objectives? We often hear people telling us from a young age, to focus but when were we actually *taught* how to do this?

These are things that you may also choose to add to your personal motivation journal for reinforcement of the types of things that you can watch out for in the future. Whether it's that long vacation in Europe or that serious mission to get yourself more physically fit, preparation of your mind is absolutely key.

"Accept the challenges, so that you may feel the exhilaration of victory."

General George S. Patton

7

GOAL-DRIVEN MOTIVATION

So, back to the previous story... Army Reserve basic training preparation. My overarching goal was to lower the amount of stress I was likely to experience during the course, by doing some forward training preparation.

Challenge accepted... but why?

Like so many people pursuing fitness objectives, I began getting tired of seeing so many books saying that it was so important to set goals. We ALREADY knew that! What is needed is to really contemplate the goal starting with the "what" and the "why". Especially the "why". If you cannot make a compelling reason to sell yourself that the goal is worthwhile, you may not achieve said goal.

My first serious training journey.

I commenced my training in the first couple of days on my vacation in Western Australia, in running shoes and shorts and t-shirt on a warm, sunny day. My end goal for training was five kilometers in twenty-six and a half minutes as per the Army Reserve requirements for my age and gender.

I really desired to achieve this during my four- week vacation where I had time, no responsibilities or regular distractions.

Day one.

On my first day of training, I jogged out slowly onto the street and then out onto the main road, which typically was a low-traffic route. It didn't take long to realize how unfit I *actually* was. After about a kilometer, I was exhausted and on the verge of throwing up. At this point, I really felt sick to my stomach and questioned what the hell I was thinking.

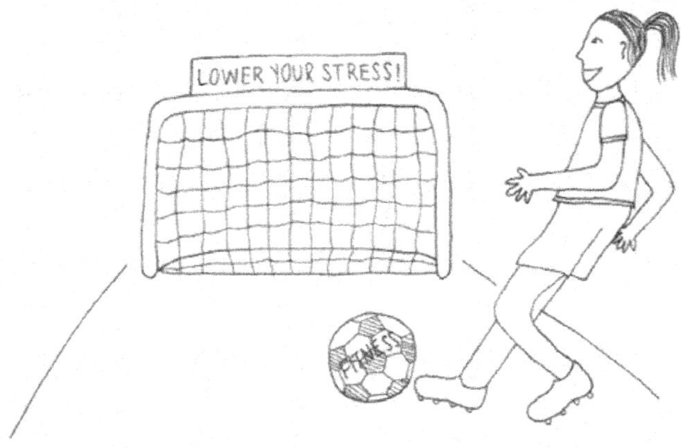

Stay on target.

After staggering back to my parents' house, I got some water and tried to mentally set aside the aching, pain and nausea. It took a couple of days, but I learned something about my motivation that surprised me. I deeply wanted to try again and this time, just for shits and giggles, I wanted to see if I could go a bit further than last time. I think that in my mind, I rationalized the bad experience as initial shock. It didn't kill me, and a battlefield would be so much worse. My intent was not to get all the way to five kilometers. I found I was able to go a little further, and even though it was painful and exhausting, I coped with it better. As days turned into weeks, I went a little further each time and even began to wear my army webbing with equipment strapped all around. I saw that by working at it more consistently and not trying for the big outcome, patience and micro changes were actually working for me. I put more emphasis on my training to be "roughly regular" more than rigidly planned, and that also seemed to help. On average I was doing a run every one to two days.

Day twenty-eight.

On my last day in Western Australia, with four hours left until my flight back to the eastern states was scheduled to leave, I had all my army equipment, full water bottles and field kits strapped to my body, in all, roughly nine kilos (or about 20 pounds). I set out for my run, and my sisters all accompanied me on their bikes. I ended up completing the five kilometers in twenty-six minutes flat. The feeling I got from that achievement was one of exhilaration and personal accomplishment. I reflected on my first attempt at running only four weeks earlier and what I was able to train myself, with my own mind, to do.

No coaching, no trainers, no prior experience, just self-monitoring and determination linked to things that I knew about myself. I also felt ready to begin training with the army, and this helped me to remove any anxiety I had about my future military training. So, if you were wondering how it went for me during my basic training course, stay tuned, more to come on that …

Takeaways? When you set out on your fitness journey, allow yourself to take it slow. Real slow. It is easier to build a habit out of something that starts as more trivial or simple than something more complex or overwhelming. It is more about training the mind into accepting a new life routine and less about building muscle. Don't worry. Over time, that will come.

CALL TO ACTION

Dig deep and think about the exercises or physical activities in your past that you really didn't enjoy. You may have tried jogging for a while or even going to a gym, or maybe it was an aerobics or CrossFit class. If these activities left you feeling tired, that just tells you that you were activating rarely used muscles and systems in your body.

Now, if an activity left you with a feeling of dread when you reminded yourself to repeat it, chances are that this mindset is an indicator that you may struggle to sustain this activity in the future.

You may also find out things about yourself that help you to overcome certain feelings or anxieties. As you begin to be reminded of things that helped you overcome a negative mindset or resistance to exercise, write these things down in your personal motivation journal.

You will have learned about your motivations through your life experiences, but you need to pull on these memories and think about how certain experiences around physical fitness affected you. You may also rediscover other things like "when I did this activity at a slower pace and gradually built it up over time, it didn't seem as challenging." Know yourself and learn from yourself.

At the right time in your journey, gyms, instructional materials and personal trainers can be *immensely* helpful to your fitness goals and provide financial self-accountability incentives and encouragement to get you motivated. However, you should try to remember that nothing you can buy or acquire replaces the value of thoughtful reflection and introspection.

*"The gem cannot be polished without friction,
nor man perfected without trials."*

CHINESE PROVERB

8

REAPING THE REWARDS FROM TRAINING YOUR MIND

About a week after returning from my vacation in Western Australia, I was feeling proud of myself and happy that I accomplished my physical preparation for military training.

February 1988.

It was time for my basic training at the recruit course for the Australian Army Reserve. I took the bus from the Australian Army Reserve Depot in Canberra to Ingleburn, NSW, where the recruit training battalion was located at Bardia Barracks. It was pretty much what I expected: corporals directing recruits, sergeants barking orders and everything rush, rush, rush. When I reflect on this, it is the way the army needs to be in order to help soldiers learn how to cope with stress, and I believe that being prepared physically was part of the formula that helped me to manage through this time.

Each day, we were woken up before 5 a.m. and put through our paces for PT, or "physical training." I was prepared to run the five kilometers with ease since there was no requirement to do it wearing loads of equipment, which was the level I had trained to. Interestingly enough, we started out on two kilometers, followed by all the other exercises mentioned in our preparation letter. While on the first two-kilometer run, I saw exactly the type of thing I wanted to avoid for myself. New recruits were stopping on the run, turning over and vomiting, heaving and breathing heavily. What made it even worse is that they were ordered to rejoin the running formation and keep going.

I was very pleased with my attitude and the effort I made in planning and preparing for this situation. To this day, I remind myself of this lesson when I have some kind of future challenge I want to meet. In addition to PT, every day was mentally demanding in the lessons we took on military protocols, badges of rank, military history, navigation, first aid, weapons, patrolling, camouflage and concealment and communications. Being fit helped me to keep myself alert and focused throughout all of the lessons. Physical toughness, strength and agility, assault courses, firing positions, and methods of movement were all significant consumers of energy just as much as practicing long hours on the parade ground learning drill formations, marching and special techniques with shouldered weapons with fixed bayonets.

I was so glad that on very limited sleep each night, I was able to meet these challenges with relative ease, especially when I could see many others who were struggling and through this, encountering the wrath of the directing staff, who were mainly junior NCOs and, in some cases, warrant officers. As our PT runs increased from two to three kilometers all the way to five, it became evident that not all people were up to the challenge, and several were "marched off" the base without being allowed to continue training and would never graduate to the status of soldier.

Among those who made it this far, a few more fell away by the time we were at the point of the ten-mile (sixteen-kilometer) forced march in boots with full battle kit and rifle. I could tell that some were either naturally fit as part of their lifestyle or, like me, had anticipated the challenges of military training and prepared themselves by following the instructions. It was the final part of our training and although it was hard, I completed it without injury or pain.

The day of the March Out Parade.

When the day of the march came, I was very fit, even more so than when I turned up. Along with all of my mates, I marched in the parade with an awesome, unbelievable sense of pride in my own accomplishments. I reflect upon that moment still to this day as a personal motivation. It helps me to remember the way I felt when I stuck to my training and did things that pushed me beyond what I thought possible. At the end, and much like the aforementioned Chinese proverb, I *did* feel like a polished gem.

Yes, there was friction, and yes, there were trials, and at the time, I was most proud of my accomplishment in passing the tests. Now, decades later, I am even more proud of my much younger self for having the intelligence and foresight in preparing my mind, preparing my body and executing flawlessly and confidently toward my goal. Proving myself to qualify for military service was great, but proving myself in terms of character, discipline and tenacity was awesome.

CALL TO ACTION

What goals have you attempted during your life? These may have been in your younger life, such as getting good grades, graduating high school or even getting your license to drive.

Goals are usually accompanied by some type of motivation or willingness that drives you to action. I can bet no one actually enjoys reading the literature on the rules of the road, but there is always a group of teenagers who have their heads buried in this text because it promises a path that will end with them in the driver's seat of a car and that translates to freedom!

Sometimes, goals are linked as a chain to achieve a highly desired outcome. To be fit, the goal should be more about what outcomes you want for yourself and less about losing fifteen pounds.

See if you can determine the real outcomes you want for yourself as far as fitness and why they are important to you. Then work out the small steps you need to create a path to success. As you begin to reflect and learn more about yourself, write these things down in your personal motivation journal to make them stick and to serve as a source of future inspiration.

"Start by doing what's necessary; then do what's possible; and suddenly you're doing the impossible."

FRANCIS OF ASSISI

9

MOTIVATIONAL TIMING

Back in 1996, I was about to do my second world trip. My adventures were to take me to the USA, Canada, Egypt, England, Wales, Nepal and Thailand. Knowing that this journey also required some physical fitness ability, especially for Egypt, Wales and Nepal, I decided to do some basic training for this endeavor. My motivation was the excitement I felt when I looked through the travel guidebooks and brochures I was studying in anticipation of this trip. Seeing pictures of Mt. Sinai in Egypt, the mountain of Pen Y Fan in Wales and the majestic peaks of the western Himalayas made me think that these would be best experienced in the most comfortable way I could muster, with a body that was physically fit and ready. This would become an example of a "motivational timing."

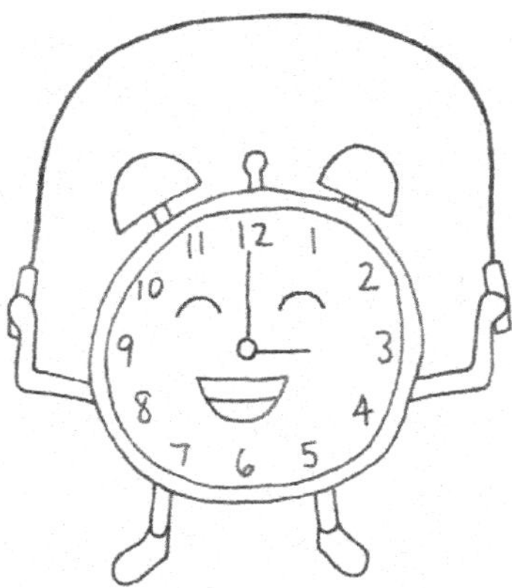

Motivational timing.

You see, I have come to think of motivational strength as something that varies according to the timing of when the motivation is applied. The motivational *timing* I used first for this adventure was "Initial Motivation." For my adventures, if I was to be able to make the effort to train, motivated with the thought of breathtaking views, memorable experiences and good health, then the training required was nonnegotiable. In the months leading up to my trip, I would take three- to five-kilometer runs, many times wearing hiking boots instead of running shoes. I would also do basics like sit-ups and push-ups for general workouts.

As the months passed, I began to slip into a routine, still fired up by the promise of exciting world travel, and it was at this point that I progressed into "Maintain Motivation." At this point, as exciting as the trip on the horizon was becoming, it was the routine and habits I had formed around training that really kept me going. Keeping this regimen up, not only conditioned my body for strenuous activity but also helped to boost my immune system, which is always a plus when traveling overseas.

All in all, the training definitely helped. I did very well with the rigor and expectations of the travel excursions and enjoyed many experiences that, unfortunately, many less prepared travelers struggled with. I saw fellow travelers in Egypt and also Nepal succumbing to the strains and physical demands of long treks, climbs and early morning starts. When I look back and consider the various times in my life when I needed motivation, I realize that my motivational "superpowers" varied from time to time, circumstance to circumstance. I used to believe that the different goals that demanded training, affected my motivation. The more captivating or alluring the goal, the more I could process this goal as a way to stimulate myself to action. What I have come to understand is that while the goals did make a difference in my motivational mindset, it was also the *stage* of my training objectives that was impactful on my motivation. I have found that motivational timing can be broken down to three stages:

Initial Motivation

This is the motivation required to *initiate* training. I have found that this is usually accompanied by feelings of excitement and positive anticipation of where the training will lead me. I have always found this being the easiest form of motivational thinking, because I have not yet had to make any physical effort or endure any physical challenges. I also believe that it is easy because of the positive feeling that I get and the improved mood I experience from the excitement at testing myself towards realizing a strategic goal or outcome.

I go through my Initial Motivation with a very positive mindset. Deciding to train intersects my love of personal challenge, the excitement of trying something new and the promise of fulfilling my future goals or outcomes. If you feel that you just cannot get your mind wrapped around wanting to begin, it might be better to delay starting a formal exercise routine and focusing on subtle habit changes instead.

Don't concern yourself with high rigor or long periods of exercise. You might even start with just a few minutes, maybe even as few as two or three, and while this may seem pointless for physical fitness, the point is to develop a mindset that begins to accept that a small amount of exercise (and therefore exercise itself) is something you can do without suffering.

You could consider other little things like parking your car further away in parking lots to force more of a walk or using the stairs for up to two flights instead of taking the elevator. You might also consider doing a few sit-ups when ads come on television or seeing what you can do when you're waiting for the oven alarm to go off while you cook something. I have done all of these things and they definitely have helped me. Little habits. Over time.

Maintain Motivation

This is the motivation required to *continue* training. I have had mixed feelings about how to approach this. Knowing that I want to continue to train has sometimes been met with personal feelings of anxiety, dread or apathy. I bet there are many people who get to this point and begin to wonder if they can keep going before feelings of dread or even guilt begin to take over and then those neural pathways begin to open up a direct passage to the "excuse" part of the brain.

We all have one and it is very powerful! When I struggle in the maintain phase, I have come to learn that for me, this is due to the memory recall of the pain, boredom or conditions that made training less of a joy and more like tedious, hard work. It is hard to ignore how something made you feel. At other times, it has been met with feelings of positive anticipation, especially in cases where I already know from past experience that the end of a training session will bring me a positive benefit like a "runner's high" or a tremendous burst of energy or a feeling of personal accomplishment.

This has always been the most difficult area of motivation for me to develop and requires self-driven commitment, dedication and a strategic value mindset. Most important of all, you really, really, really need to know your feelings, your mood and actually ask yourself how you want to work through it. Maybe you need to slow it down. Maybe you need to re-affirm the benefits it will bring. Maybe you just need to say to yourself, "for the next 10 minutes, I can at *least* do this."

A strategic value mindset is more about focusing on a point in the future and thinking about what you want that point in time to be like in terms of your health and overall physical abilities. It can be challenging, especially when the tactical side of your brain can shut any strategic value argument down with a whole range of excuses for why *not* to exercise.

Remember my earlier remark about that "excuse area of the brain". Yes, I definitely made that up but, you have to admit, it's pretty powerful! Maintain Motivation has definitely always been the hardest for me to conquer. I have learned several techniques that work with my mindset that make it easier for me to manage and continue.

For example, I am a firm believer that some training continuously is better than scattered bursts of training. I also accept that on some days, I will *not* be doing quite the same rigor as the day before, whether it is time on the elliptical, the weight of the dumbbells or the reps in my floor exercises.

This was something that took me a long time to come to accept. I was always taught or shown that you had to do a certain number or meet a certain time or be a certain level of ability but in the end, I have grown to accept that these numbers do not account for personal circumstances, feelings or the psyche of the individual.

So, for me, I have the honor system. Did I commit and follow through on doing *something* instead of nothing? Did I make an effort or wander off and watch cat-videos on Facebook? I only have myself to answer in the end. The main thing is that now, with my *maintain* motivation pretty much intact, I continue to train five to six days a week and that I always break a sweat and activate the muscle groups, especially my core.

You may find that maintaining motivation is easier if you have a personal trainer, and I believe they provide an enormous amount of value to learning and applying good techniques while cheering you on and pushing you further. I have been fortunate to have worked with some great personal trainers who bring variety, knowledge and patience to help you get through your workouts. They also understand body mechanics which is so essential for form and for physical safety.

Reset Motivation

This is a combination of Initial and Maintain Motivation. It is the motivation required to *get back on track* in training after suspension of activity or an unavoidable life setback. A suspension of activity may be something like a significant injury or surgery where medical advice has been given to suspend training. An unavoidable life setback might be extended travel arrangements, a death in the family or a setback with employment or livelihood. Reset Motivation can be like Initial Motivation because you feel like you are beginning all over again. The main difference is that you have stored memories of accomplishing a regular routine of fitness in the past.

Reset Motivation can, however, be delayed when there are feelings of guilt from not exercising for an extended period of time. One of the strategies I use to tackle Reset Motivation is to remind myself that I DID get into a routine in the past and that I made it continuous and habitual. When I remind myself of this, I am energized to "get back in the saddle" and to feel like I can rebuild my routine. I also prepare myself with reasonable expectations like choosing *not* to expect myself to reenter training to the same level as where I suspended it. I know it is wiser to restart a little slower and a little less aggressively than before even—and this is very important—even if I feel like I *could* do more. The reason is that I need to condition my mind back into a routine and at the start, this is actually more important than conditioning my body. Be kind to yourself and allow a little time to readjust.

CALL TO ACTION

Initial Motivation.

Consider the types of things or factors that help to get you started on a journey. Consider your present circumstances. What is achievable and what is necessary to get started?

Maintain Motivation.

What keeps you going? What do you know about yourself that makes it hard to stick to things? What do you need to tell yourself or to remind yourself of?

Reset Motivation.

What helps you to "get back in the saddle"? If circumstances change for you—a job loss, a family circumstance—how will you cope? Do you have a network of people to help you? Do you know things about yourself that you can draw on from past experiences to re-use?

It is necessary to think about these things as you develop your abilities to start, sustain and reset your motivation for fitness.

Now, just write it.

As you explore your inner experiences and the things that make you tick, write down these discoveries in your Personal Motivation Journal.

These discoveries can help you develop more insightful approaches to the motivations you wish to master, whether it is to begin your journey, maintain your progress or press the reset button and start over.

"Obstacles don't have to stop you. If you run into a wall, don't turn around and give up. Figure out how to climb it, go through it, or work around it."

Michael Jordan

10

SELF-DISCIPLINE IS HARD: IT'S ALL ON YOU

Many years ago, I was out shopping with my daughter Cassie. She was ten or eleven years old. During that afternoon, we took an unplanned detour into a shoe store. Not for any particular reason—just to browse. Cassie was clutching onto her twenty dollars she had saved from her allowances, and she soon began looking at shoes that interested her.

Strange as it may seem, life lessons can be found in many different situations and circumstances. I never thought that walking into a shoe store would lead to something that would help with training the mind!

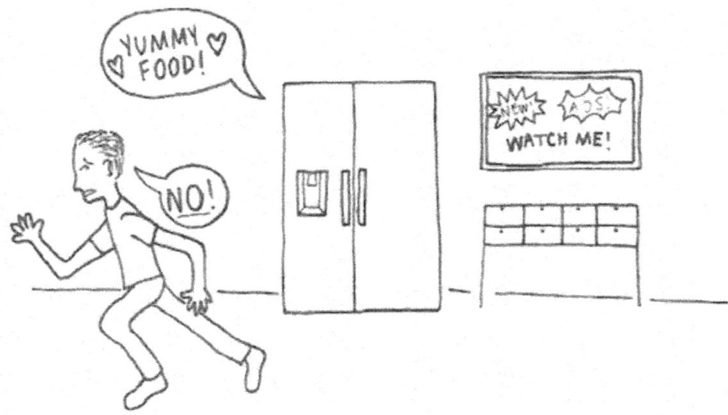

Temptations, leave me alone!

After a little browsing, she found a pair of very cool shoes. She loved the style, she loved how they felt on her feet and she loved the teal color they came in. By this time, she was about ready to buy them since she had enough money, but wasn't sure, because it meant she would have no money left and she feared that if she saw something else she wanted or needed later, she would not have enough money. She wanted to have the self-discipline to leave the store, but she also wanted to be good with her decision and not feel like she passed up a good opportunity. The answer lay at her feet and was inside her; she just needed to look inside and find it. A teachable moment to train the mind!

I went up to Cassie and suggested that she should close her eyes for about thirty seconds and then *imagine* how she would have felt about her day later, if she had never even walked into the shoe store. As if we never took that detour and she never browsed any racks of new and colorful shoes. After thirty seconds of thinking, Cassie opened her eyes, put the shoes back on the rack and said, "let's go." She never even gave the shoes a second thought. This showed her that if something was difficult to decide or that a desire was testing her mental discipline, she just needed to do some inner searching to find the answer. It didn't even take that long.

Introspection is key.

Thoughtful introspection to explore your desires, your needs and your feelings is a tool that is forever useful for helping you to discover *what* things are important to you, *why* they are important to you and *how* you want to proceed. How many times have you heard people say, "all that is needed is some good ol' self-discipline"? I plead guilty in having said this myself, in the past. Self-discipline is the act of motivating yourself to do things that you may not be ready to do or even *want* to do. Where integrity is doing the right thing when no one else is looking, self-discipline is doing the necessary things when no one else is pushing. Self-discipline is a test of your personal will, your strength of conviction and your confidence in yourself to do the hard things.

Excuses burn zero calories.

Excuses can be the enemy of self-discipline. Of course, in life many excuses are valid, and life throws so many things our way, that things like exercise are easy to deprioritize, but many times we are tempted to overplay the urgency or severity of an excuse. Again, it all comes back to how well you really know yourself and how honest you want to be in admitting your personal shortcomings or challenges. Your shortcomings and challenges are nothing to necessarily be embarrassed about, but it is important to own up to them so that you can work them into your mindset. Part of your mindset will always be that part of you that wants to do the easier thing more than the harder thing. When you see a path forward with a fork in the road that can take you toward easier things or more challenging things, you can very easily and creatively come up with excuses as to why you should do the easier thing. This is why the mind benefits from training.

We are very influential on ourselves and if we allow it, we can win every argument as we debate the path we take and the decisions we make. When you find yourself conflicted between that part of yourself that argues the need for you to do exercise and that part of you that finds reasons why you cannot, it can be easier for the latter to win the argument. In the end, the argument you win is always with yourself and you may satisfy yourself with the decision you made in your own mind because you listened to "reason", even though it was still you.

Typically, where exercise is concerned, the excuses are universal. "I don't have enough time in the day" is one of the more popular ones. The day is filled with twenty-four hours, and unless you cannot fit in a couple of ten-minute exercise bursts in a twenty-four-hour period, having no time is not really an excuse. "I have injuries." Yes, this could indeed have a profound impact on being able to exercise, but the thing to remember is that you may be able to engage in *some* activity in certain areas of your body. "I am too old." Unless some mental or physical barrier prevents exercise or puts you at risk of injury, being of a certain age should be something you consider carefully and assess whether it is really valid. Another conversation with your physician can hardly hurt either. "I am too big." Sometimes the size of our bodies can be a barrier to movement, and I believe in some of these cases, it is important to consider that even the smallest of exercises beats doing nothing. Everyone's physical limitations and circumstances are different, so motivating yourself with this knowledge in mind, is essential to approaching any exercise in safety.

Certainly, the goal would be to slowly build upon the small things and gradually make things more rigorous. "Exercise is difficult." I think that the best thing I can say to this excuse is "no duh!" The last excuse, and I know there are more, is this: "I will do it … but later." Procrastination is something that you have to acknowledge as an aspect of your personality before you can begin to address it. At the end of the day, know that excuses will inevitably present themselves from time to time and recognize that self-discipline is something that you can develop and use to counter most if not all of the invalid or BS excuses. Also remember that it takes time and if it helps, ask others to keep you committed to your goals.

CALL TO ACTION

Present yourself with a challenge of self-discipline that keeps you accountable to something you are willing to do. *Before* undertaking any physical challenge, first take some time to ask yourself some probing questions in order to gain an insight as to the likelihood of success. Be honest.

Don't worry when you are thinking; nobody is looking.

Here are some questions to ask yourself:

If I am a procrastinator, what excuses typically block me from acting in a timely manner? What is the minimum amount of activity that I think I can actually commit to?

If I cannot hold myself accountable to the action I know I need to take, who or what can keep me accountable? Think about this carefully and then set yourself up with a challenge to exercise that self-discipline muscle! The goal is to see what level of self-discipline you are willing to tackle and see it through to the end. Be careful, though. If you pick something that is unachievable, this may become very *demotivational* to you, so pick something you know you can do, and more importantly, are *willing* to do.

To make sure you execute on this goal, I suggest giving yourself a time frame of a week. Here are some examples that you may consider or use to spark your own ideas.

Before I eat a big meal, what activity can I safely do that can burn a few calories in a short amount of time?

When I am sitting in front of the television and an ad comes on, what can I safely do during the commercial break or even for a single ad?

Is there a relative or friend I can spend some time with or connect with over a safe physical activity? Take some time to record what you learn and discover in your personal motivation journal.

"Do something every day that you don't want to do. This is the golden rule of acquiring the habit of doing your duty without pain."

Mark Twain

11

MAKING IT STICK

A few years ago, I began developing slight discomfort in my lower back, and this spread into sciatica pain down my legs and finally became more severe with every passing day. I consulted my physician, who examined me and gave me muscle relaxants. The muscle relaxants did make a slight difference, but soon the pain returned. My doctor reexamined me and put me on a course of painkillers that I could take as needed. The painkillers had limited and inconsistent impact, and after a few weeks, the pain got progressively worse until one day as I tried to swivel off the side of my bed, I suddenly experienced severe lower back pain to the point where I could barely stand up or walk.

My partner took me to the emergency room and my kids were noticeably concerned as I departed the house. My partner was also concerned, as was I. After consulting with the emergency room physician and discussing the various treatments I had tried using, the physician prescribed another round of muscle relaxants and then told me one simple and clear sentence: "You just have to fix your core." I immediately thought about this insight and in a split second, I realized that this made complete sense. We had talked about my age, my lifestyle and my vitals, and working on my core made sense, at the very least, as something I should try.

The details beyond this are interesting in terms of the actions I took to make changes, especially when confronted by the possibilities of back therapy, stronger medication and even surgery. Suffice it to say, I took steps to get to a point where I could begin training to improve my core, as per the good doctor's advice.

The outcome from all of this was that on self-inspection, the two things that motivated me very highly were the wake-up call about the state of my health and the advice of the doctor. The doctor's comment actually inspired my initial motivation to get fit, and the thought of getting my core in shape was the kind of challenge that someone with *my* personality would embrace. However, this would never be lasting and so it was really the wake-up call about the state of my health that gave me the staying power to making my training stick, something I have developed, expanded and maintained to this very day.

Initiating training can be brought on or stimulated by an immediate need, a new idea or something that looks appealing. People may become excited at the thought of a highly discounted home gym advertised on television, or the sight of treadmills in a suburban store, or even the prospect of an event that inspires them look good for that special occasion, maybe a school reunion or a wedding.

This initial motivation is usually the easy part, but it is nonetheless essential to begin the journey. During this initial training phase, it may be a good idea to question the motivation for action in terms of how long you want your training to last and under what terms. Would you want it to last right until the special event you are excited about? Would you want to do it until that home gym is fully paid off? Do you look at training as important to your body image and your overall health, or even as a more lasting lifestyle choice to create a more positive future for yourself in terms of your health and overall abilities?

No matter what answers you arrive at, you may arrive at a place where you begin training, even if it is something that you're not sure you'll maintain, enjoy or even be capable of. You may find yourself beginning a training routine after a while. It may not be perfectly regimented or even enjoyable, but you still want to try and keep going, even if you are motivated by feelings of guilt about giving in, by trying to keep yourself challenged or because you innately know it's the right thing for your overall and future well-being.

Lifestyle habits.

Once you have hit a certain stride or rhythm in your training, it is important not to take those days or weeks in a row for granted. Making it stick is all about taking a routine and making it into a lifestyle habit. It is said and widely believed that it usually takes doing something for a month continuously, to make a new behavior into a habit. Habits can sometimes be bad, but they can also be very good. Every morning, we habitually follow some type of routine, from the time we first stir from our slumber to the time we exit the house to go to work, out to run errands or go to school. Habits feel less like work and more like you are doing activities on autopilot. If there is a way to introduce some exercise into an already established routine, it may be habit forming and easier for you to sustain.

If your schedule allows you more flexibility in the evening, then see which evenings may give you the most flexibility. It might be a walk, it might be a quick visit to the gym on the way home from work, it might be dropping by the community center just to have a go at the climbing wall. Make it something you feel you can do regularly and is less likely to be impacted by the other demands and responsibilities of your day-to-day life. Exercise doesn't have to be high rigor. Making it stick is easier if you feel less overwhelmed to go and do some activity and in your own time, you may choose to increase the time, the intensity or the repetitions while you vary the activities to keep it interesting.

Running into issues.

I learned early in life that running is an effective fitness activity for me. It helps me develop leg strength and cardiovascular endurance and moderates my weight. The trouble for me with running is that I learned that for me, it is unsustainable. For one thing, I had already had two knee surgeries on my right knee, so running on hard surfaces wasn't very good for it. The bigger reason for running being unsustainable was that it was tedious and boring. I did try playing an MP3 playlist of hard rock songs and this helped a little, but I was still bored and I felt more like I was doing something that was mentally pointless and uninteresting.

The only time running was interesting for me was when I set a goal of completing a half marathon in the year of my fortieth birthday. Having a running partner and a set goal in mind made it far more interesting and sustainable. More about how I trained my mind to train for the half marathon in another chapter, so stay tuned. I guess the thing that I learned is that if you find the right mix of factors that can make something more sustainable, it is worth at least trying. A smaller effort can make it easier on the mind as well as the body too. Where it comes to training my own mind toward finding activities that stick, I reexamine the things that I know, believe and have learned about myself. Oh, and by the way, these attributes have changed as I have advanced through different stages of my life.

For example, I know that things are easier for me to sustain if they are more accessible. For the longest time, I never had a workout room in my basement, but in my earlier life, I had a vehicle at my disposal, that made going to the gym more accessible. As my life changed through employment, marriage and parenthood, suddenly the gym wasn't always as accessible as it had once been, even though I had a better vehicle. So, I learned that, for me, accessibility isn't just about overcoming distance; it is also about being able to maximize my time.

Repurposing mis-spent time.

When I realized that watching television was a way to help me relax, I found that I had an intense dislike for commercials. Not because they were disrupting my show—I know they are a necessary part of funding commercial television works—but because of the increasing length of commercials and the intelligence-insulting messaging that mass media marketing directs toward its audience. It was the true embodiment of wasting my time in ways I could not stand. With a little imagination, I worked out that I could repurpose that time by doing light exercises.

Sometimes it would be a set of push-ups or sit-ups, other times it would be neck stretches while seated or light yoga poses on the floor in front of the television.

Other efforts I chose often involved doing some productive and yet active core that got me out of my seat and also helped me to accomplish some neglected household tasks. I learned making things more accessible is one thing, but providing some additional benefit or finding ways to maximize otherwise wasted time were techniques that I could sustain. Try using some introspection to find the things that drive you to action, then use your imagination to discover the types of activities you are more likely to do.

CALL TO ACTION

What are the things about yourself that you know, have learned or have experienced that are more likely to make an activity stick? In your personal motivation journal, write down a few things that can help make an activity stick.

Here are some examples to get you thinking:

If the activity is inexpensive or free, I am more likely to do it because money is not a barrier.

I prefer less complicated activities that do not require special equipment. If the activity fits within my own physical limitations, I am more likely to keep it up.

I don't have much time. I look for things that can be done in ten minutes or less.

Activities that help me get things done while burning calories can become a double positive for me.

Having fun at something makes me more likely to stick with it. Great music makes me want to dance.

I need something that incorporates learning technical skills, like martial arts. I know that exercising by myself can be lonely, so who can I be active with?

I get my energy from sunshine and being outdoors. Nice days are not always available, but something is better than nothing. I like the occasional TV binge watch, but a few leg raises and arm raises through the commercials might be something I can try from time to time when safe to do so.

Which of these apply to you? What other things not on this list may also apply?

Take a few moments and write these things down in your personal motivation journal.

"The only place where success comes before work is in the dictionary."

Vidal Sassoon

12

DOING NOTHING BURNS ZERO CALORIES

In the past few years, the intensity of my fitness routines has increased to a fairly good level for someone my age. I was once asked if I am looking to extend my level of intensity and ability to even higher levels, and the question gave me pause to really look inside of myself and my inner attitudes to find the answer. I wondered if my morning routine that comprises a five-minute medium-intensity elliptical cardio warm-up, followed by two hundred mixed exercise reps mostly for core, followed by three hundred mixed reps for strength and flexibility and then a warm down with a few minutes of planks could be extended further. The answer I arrived at was interesting.

I do enough regular exercise and at sustained regularity that I do not have to increase reps, or weights, or even levels of elliptical machine resistance to extend anything. The interesting thing is that if I can maintain these levels of intensity, reps and weights going forward, the only thing that has to change is my age. Every day that I maintain these exercises, I am, over time, burning calories and improving my health with a slightly older body.

By the way, there is a bonus chapter in this book that covers some insights on varying levels of workout intensity!

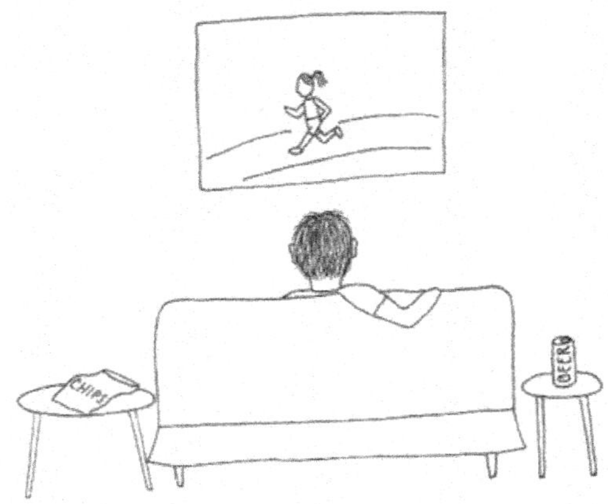

TV, chips and beer – ugh.

My age changing is, in itself, an extender of my workouts by default. Some may disagree with this assessment, but for me, and maybe for you, it may make sense. I think you have to first find what level you want to reach and then consider if you want to extend it further in the ways that make most sense to you. The bottom line is this: "Doing nothing burns zero calories!"

There will be times when you just do *not* want to do anything. It will be tempting to think that the worst part of this is the fact that you will not do your workout and keep your commitment to yourself. Putting this kind of pressure on yourself does little to give you credit for the activity you have already achieved. Once you feel this self-imposed pressure it becomes easier to seed self-doubt and lead yourself down a path of diminishing commitment. If you make less and less time for yourself, you may begin to associate your doubt and guilt for stopping with the act of exercise itself.

This is what many people tend to slip into and what makes it worse is that in the future, that motivation to reengage is already being met with the memory of the guilt and disappointment from past experiences. This is why this book is all about training the mind first, in order to become better at training the body. The minute we lose focus on the importance of training the mind, it becomes more difficult to continuously train the body.

A better alternative to consider would be one that looks at physical activity and well-being as more about the journey and less about the destination. Setting your mind to be more accepting of a more lasting journey that contains ups and downs is healthier. The commitment to focus is one continuous activity, and over time, the intensity and higher levels of progress will come. Give it some time, but keep going.

Momentum is key. Even when you're not "feeling it," think of some things that can still be beneficial. Gentle stretches, easier yoga positions, finding a quiet place and focusing on your breathing all contribute to remarkable health benefits. They can also be used as a bridge between more rigorous workouts for the days when you are set and motivated for higher intensity and your head is more in the game. Even during the workout, you may find that you just don't want to go through certain levels of intensity. When this happens, give yourself some credit for starting and for the exercise already completed. If you need a rest, then rest, and if you prefer to rest while still working out, find something milder like stretching or isometrics that gives you a chance to do less while maintaining some value.

Fitness instructors have a name for this: "active recovery." When I used to run for fitness, I applied a similar principle, where I would set small goals to run a small distance and then walk a small distance. I used to call my method "run-walking" but later I was to find out that runners referred to this with the term interval-training. It can be fun to try out new techniques and even though my methods were things I made-up, I found that through experimentation, some actually worked. Coincidentally, I found out later that these methods were already known and proven in wider fitness circles, just defined with different names.

As with many things in life, knowing how your motivation works begins with digging deep and truly exploring yourself and understanding what makes you happy, frustrated, energized or accomplished. It does not happen in a specific time; it happens as you try to understand yourself more thoroughly and honestly. In psychology, Maslow's hierarchy of needs treats this as reaching "self-actualization." Once you begin to understand your true self, you will work out what it takes to get you from couch to crunch and create the will to move more than to remain motionless. When you stay moving, the benefit is more than what the exercise does for your body, it is also the benefit you get from keeping your mind trained to maintain physical activity as a habit that becomes a lifestyle.

Safety first.

As with all activities, ensure that you take care of your physical safety and that of those around you first. Try not to attempt those handstands in the living room when your children are around! Be careful in rooms where you have heavy workout machinery or treadmills and elliptical machines, especially if there is the chance that a child or pet may wander in to your workout space. For yourself, always make sure that you have consulted with your physician to understand the things that you should and should not do. Doing something that brings about a severe injury not only defeats the purpose of becoming healthier but it also presents itself as a setback that you first have to recover from in order to reset your motivation.

CALL TO ACTION

As we get older, time can seem to accelerate at an even faster pace and we also seem to have less of it. Each passing day, you can reflect upon and ask yourself some questions in order to assess the things you could have done even if time or circumstances presented constraints.

Dig deep and consider the following passages and write down your comments in your personal motivation journal.

Describe any time when you could have done some safe exercises for three to five minutes.

Consider any opportunity during your lunch break when you might be able to do some short walks.

When you find yourself sitting down, ask yourself "could I do some seated gentle isometric exercises or stretches for my neck, arms or shoulders?"

"Those who wish to sing, always find a song."

Swedish Proverb

13

FUN IS ALWAYS A GOOD MOTIVATOR

In recent years, I have observed the emerging technology for fun that we are seeing in our smartphones, tablets and watches. One of the things I observed, that my kids got me interested in was connected to a kind of hobby that my son, Mattie, loved: Pokémon. Mattie loved everything about Pokémon from the cards, the toys, the movies, the video games and the conversations we would have about collecting all things connected to this vast and thriving Japanese creature universe. The well-known battle cry for Pokémon is "gotta catch 'em all," and this concept was the basis for a fairly sophisticated scavenger hunt made for mobile devices called "Pokémon Go."

Gotta catch 'em!

Essentially, the game puts you in the role of a Pokémon trainer who has to physically travel to and through places around the world in order to find and collect Pokémon using a virtual reality viewer. This game made a fun concept like the scavenger hunt simple and easy, and it was fun to go for walks in the hope of finding and adding more Pokémon to your collection.

Since this provided an activity that I could enjoy with my kids, I took to this opportunity like a duck to water, and we all went Pokémon collecting together, always comparing our finds and their particular point levels and helping each other in battling our Pokémon against other trainers in virtual gyms that we would have to walk and navigate to. It became such a fun activity that I took to doing long walks during my lunch break. I was soon to find out that a whole group of grown adults at my work campus were also in on this new game, and we all soon became friends, caught Pokémon and did a LOT of walking!

Since that time, I have also discovered other things for fun, My continuous life-long-learning and curiosity for so many topics makes it hard to find the time to feed my mind. I had heard about audiobooks and podcasts for many years, but never felt compelled to listen to them inside the home with all of its normal distractions and responsibilities. So, I thought, what about listening to audiobooks on my smartphone while walking? Soon, from audiobooks, I was soon extending that interest to downloading TED talk videos and podcasts that have provided learning items and general topics of interest that help me enjoy my long walks without ever feeling bored. In fact, there are times I wish I had more time to just *keep* walking! The main thing I learned is that if you can incorporate something that makes you feel like you are having fun or doing something satisfying for yourself while committing to some type of activity, it is an opportunity not to be missed.

Lifestyle habits.

Once you have hit a certain stride or rhythm in your exercise routine, it is always helpful to find ways to make the activity even more enjoyable. I need mental stimulation for exercise that at times, can be a little mundane, which for me is walking or jogging. Music playlists on my phone and podcasts of interesting topics are very helpful to me; the podcasts in particular also help me to learn new things or explore new ideas. You may also download great treasure hunt-style applications for your phone.

Of course, for me, nothing really beats nice weather and pleasant scenery. Many times, the exercise itself can be a fun activity. For fun, I think my favorite is probably rappelling. If you like dancing and dancing is what will get you in the mood to move your body, stretch your limbs and get your blood pumping, you can take classes that incorporate dance as a form of exercise. If you work with a personal trainer in a gym, see if they are open to letting you submit a playlist during your workout or finding music that can be used to time certain exercise routines. I often use certain songs for different types of workouts based on intensity, especially when I need that adrenalin surge that helps me to push myself along with the beat and rhythms of heavy rock!

If you have a workout room in your home, make it suit how you can focus and feel comfortable and even inspired to give it your all. Sometimes a TV may be a good thing to have just so you can be exercising while watching the morning news, or if you have an older tablet like an iPad that you no longer need, you can use it as a movie player on your treadmill or elliptical machine. The one thing that many people do with the home workout area in their basement is to leave it surrounded by junk, and this is probably not the ideal setting to help you focus on your fitness goals. Maybe a workout area is just the inspiration you need to clear out some space and maybe even get rid of a few items. Never be afraid of deleting some of that clutter!

If you are lucky enough to have a space, something about ten feet by ten feet would be ample. You really do not *need* to get all of those big gym machines or apparatuses if you want to stay in shape. Hand weights, a stability ball, an aerobic step with a few extra height extenders, resistance bands and exercise mats will get you going in no time. Take that old boom box you never really used and repurpose it for your gym! If you have boring walls, dress them up with inspirational messages or posters of things that help you develop a sense of mission toward your exercise goals. I am not suggesting that you go out and purchase every poster for all the Rocky films or photos of Arnie, but if you think something visual and striking will help, then go for it.

I remember staying in an apartment community a while back and I will never forget how they decorated the workout room in posters of all of these sickeningly fancy desserts. I wasn't sure about the point they were trying to make. Maybe it was if you exercise you can go crazy and eat all of this junk? The mystery continues. You may even want to think about the people you have in your life, and they may inspire you to be in better shape for their sake. You can always place family photos around your workout area.

CALL TO ACTION

As we change through ages and through the phases of our life, our notion of fun also changes. The things that were fun when you were younger may no longer be as appealing or as satisfying as they were in the past, and the things that feel like fun to you now may not have been thought of as "fun" to your twentysomething self.

Now might be a good time to consider the things that you now see as more like fun that you can also connect to an activity that gets you motivated to exercise.

Have a think about how you may be able to setup some workout space in your home. It may be an area in your living room, it may be a lower level or even an outdoor patio if you have great weather.

Try and list a few things in your personal motivation journal that are fun, safe and achievable to your present-day self that will also help you burn a few calories on a regular or even semi-regular basis.

If you can think of a few things, it will give you some variety. Most people do not even give this concept a moment's consideration, but I have faith in you that if you really think it through carefully, you may find things that you like to do, learn or try out that could make exercise a by-product of having fun.

"All the adversity I've had in my life, all my troubles and obstacles, have strengthened me … You may not realize it when it happens, but a kick in the teeth may be the best thing in the world for you."

Walt Disney

14

SETBACKS HAPPEN: LEARN TO WORK THROUGH AND IN SPITE OF THEM

In 2004, I realized I was headed toward my fortieth birthday, and I set myself a personal challenge to see what my forty-year-old self was capable of. I decided to enter into a challenge that was physically demanding, something I had not actually done before, and this turned out to be the state-to-state half marathon, 13.1 miles of distance crossing from Ohio into Indiana and back again. I trained with a friend for several months all the time, gaining in strength, determination and endurance. I remember that at the point in my training where I was almost ready, I did a ten-mile community fun run and actually placed third in my age group. Don't worry about cheering, there were only three in my age group!

Not long after that, I was training on a seven-miler and my right knee, which had a history of problems, was getting very sore and irritated to the point of intense pain. I stopped at about the two-mile mark and rested until I could drive home and consider my predicament. I was distraught about what this might mean for my half marathon coming up in about six weeks. I decided to fight my inner concerns and rest up for about five days in order to give my knee a chance to recover and to keep my mind from dwelling on this situation. After five days of this setback, I went on a three-mile run and I felt fine. Soon after, I was back on track and went on to complete the half marathon comfortably and without injury. I learned from that experience that with setbacks, it is perhaps better to acknowledge them and allow yourself some time for your mind and body to be calm and then get back into it with renewed vigor.

One of the most frustrating things that can occur in your fitness journey are setbacks. Not only do setbacks stall your progress, they mess with your mind and make you begin to have thoughts of doubt, guilt or worry that may make it hard to "get back on the wagon." Setbacks can occur at any time and for any reasons, especially reasons that are outside of your control. Life is largely unpredictable, and as a human being on this planet, no matter who you are, how much wealth or power you have amassed or what your abilities may be, you will always experience things that throw a wrench in the machinery of good intentions and commitments.

A very basic and yet understandable setback to sustaining fitness activities is injury or illness. I have experienced injuries during long-term physically demanding commitments for training, and it was very frustrating because it felt like things beyond my control were interfering with my hard work and self-discipline. I had to understand and accept that we are not always in the best of health. Our attitude toward how we handle injuries and illness during and after will make a big difference in our fitness lifestyle.

It may become very easy to feel disappointed or even a little guilty about letting yourself down, but this really is something that you should strive to avoid. The most valuable thing I learned about myself throughout my journey is that it is healthier to cultivate an understanding and acceptance that setbacks are a natural and even expected part of a training journey. I wish that someone had told me that when I was much younger. Instead of chastising myself for setbacks and building concern around my ability to continue, it would have been less stressful to accept the setback and then stop. Breathe. Regroup. Remind yourself that injury and illness, unless very severe, are in many cases nothing more than a temporary state of affairs. Take your time, heal and then get back into it, slowly at first.

Look to the examples of people in our society who have overcome physical adversity to become the most incredible people you will ever hear about and take some inspiration from them. Rick Allen is the drummer of Def Leppard who in 1984 had his entire left arm amputated and has continued to drum for the band with a single hand to this day. Malala Yousafzai is a Pakistani woman who was shot in the head as a young girl and who has become one of the world's foremost speakers and influencers on women's issues in cultures that negatively impact women. What we can learn from these people isn't just that they had the grit and determination to overcome such severe setbacks, but also that they were able to know enough about themselves to recognize the things that would motivate them to move mountains, not just obstacles. This would not have been easy, but having the right mindset built their confidence, and their will to survive is surely something to aspire to.

CALL TO ACTION

We all encounter setbacks in our lives. Some occur due to things outside of our control, some things occur due to things inside someone else's control or influence, and some things occur outside anybody's control!

Setbacks can deeply affect the steady, sustained and maintained motivation you have cultivated toward your fitness journey. Setbacks are usually inevitable and almost always frustrating. It is important to *accept* that setbacks can and will most likely occur. Life is largely unpredictable so get used to it. Then, *prepare* for it. *Train* your mind to accept setbacks and then *use* your mind to overcome them. It is up to you to manage them so that you can get back into your fitness routines.

In your personal motivation journal, write down the things that you can do or call upon that will help you prevent or manage the setbacks over which you have more control.

Follow that up with some personal motivation insights about how you need to think and act when setbacks outside your control affect your fitness journey.

"The man who dares to waste one hour of time has not discovered the value of life."

CHARLES DARWIN

15

WE FIND TIME FOR THE THINGS THAT MATTER

A few years ago, I was in a radiologist's waiting room waiting to have my hand x-rayed after fairly rigorous board breaking at martial arts training. I was also training to learn and execute a new kick—the two-step-jump-side kick. I knew that my flexibility needed a little upgrading, and I was trying to find time to work on my hamstring and calf stretches. While I was in the waiting room and after being told that the wait was going to be a while, I decided to guard my injured hand and focus on doing all my leg stretches right there in the waiting room, using the floor and even my chair for the stretches. To me it didn't matter because there was only one other person with me in the room watching television. After about ten minutes, more patients began arriving and filling up the room, but not to capacity. I figured I would just keep going because it was effectively using the time and not allowing the anxiety of waiting get to me. In fact, after a good thirty minutes of various stretches and light exercises, I was more relaxed and of course limber. The lesson learned for me was this. If you really want to, you can always find time for the things that matter, but you have to want to do it.

Life is busy whether you are a student, an office worker, a parent or even taking a vacation. Time to invest in exercise can be difficult to find. But is it really? One of the most common reasons I hear from people struggling with getting fit is that they have no time or not enough. As we pass through each phase of our life, we become entangled with different activities and responsibilities that make grabs for our time. School. Family, Work. Household chores. Financial management. Relationships. Health. Unfortunately, health takes a very customary back seat and low order in the way we prioritize our actions and the choices we make in how we use time. There is much more time than we allow ourselves to believe, but we need to either find it or create it.

FSO and GSD

Many people are consumed with their full-time work and allow themselves to be constant workaholics. Performing office heroics rarely gets you credit and only robs you of the time you need for yourself. You need to figure out ways to escape that. It isn't always easy to say no to your boss or to take a risk and find a new job, but a little FSO (figuring shit out) always goes a long way. I like to think of FSO as the precursor to the action I call GSD (getting shit done).

When we find wasted time, we need to figure out how to be more productive. If you are in a doctor's waiting room, you can make use of that time. Administrative things take time at home like paying bills or teaching yourself things you need to learn by discreetly watching online videos or listening to podcasts. Basically, if you need time for something, figure out where you can be more efficient because at the end of it all, you will release some time and that time can be repurposed to focus on your health.

Each workday is filled with twenty-four hours. If we commit ten hours to sleep, hygiene and meals, with another ten for working and commuting, that leaves four hours. For people working two or more jobs or for folks with much longer commute times, the time is easily eroded, and I have also been victim of those circumstances. Naturally we live according to our circumstances, and careful and constant introspection is often necessary to figure out how you may best adjust your circumstances, beginning with things you can control. If you work too many hours but you tend to use escalators or elevators at work, then you may be able to repurpose some of that elevator wait and operating time and take the stairs, especially for short journeys.

Time can be an easy thing to waste and under-value. The older we get, the faster it seems to pass. The framework I created below can help you train your mind to become better at how you can become better in finding time to help you stay motivated.

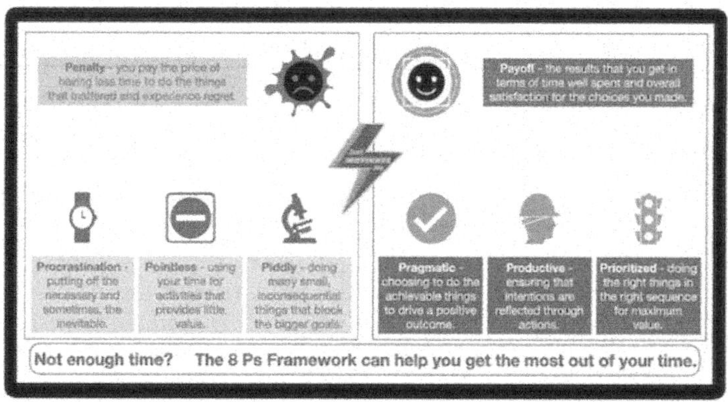

The 8 P's Framework for thoughtfully using time.

When you finally figure out how to reclaim time for yourself, determine how you best want to use it. Your family, your spouse and your health are a good start. Or you might say: "I also need some mental downtime to watch some TV." You may say that you need to take in some books for self-study or self-indulgence. Exercise is also and almost always an option too! Try out the 8 Ps framework for evaluating the use of your time.

CALL TO ACTION

Spend some time to *find* more time. You may have heard the saying "you have to spend money to make money." This is very similar. We can allow ourselves to believe that the time we need will just show up. When the time presents itself, we have rarely planned an effective use for it. Try this.

Get some time to yourself. You can do it. I believe in you. Say fifteen to thirty minutes, and grab your personal motivation journal to write in. Look at it like writing a budget, but instead of determining where you spend money, use it to determine where you spend time.

Think of time spent waiting, for instance, in waiting rooms, bus stops or train stations. How could you use that time better? Perhaps you can go through email, clear out old contacts, complete administrative tasks or reconnect with people via text. Maybe you can do some neck stretches or focused breathing exercises. Write down what you come up with. Think of times you spend idle like riding the bus or train to work. Maybe you have vacation or sick days you can use. I know that even when I am hanging around airport departure lounges, I prefer to be doing some stretches rather than just sitting around.

What could be useful to you? Catch up on some learning objectives or research better deals for your phone or internet services. Maybe some seated isometrics are possible. Write down what you come up with. Think of times when you are frustrated by wasted time. You see commercial after commercial on television taking more and more of your viewing time and insulting your intelligence all at the same time.

Could you repurpose that time to being active and getting some "micro chores" done? Rinse the dishes, collect the trash around the house, make a shopping list. On large commercial breaks, go find the vacuum cleaner and maybe do a room or two. You get a cleaner home and some exercise all at once. Whatever you determine, yes, you know the drill by now … Write it down. Once you have written these things down, revisit them along with all of the other personal insights to help you in your journey.

"There is a saying in Tibetan, 'Tragedy should be utilized as a source of strength.' No matter what sort of difficulties, how painful experience is, if we lose our hope, that's our real disaster."

DALAI LAMA XIV

16

GETTING THROUGH THE GUILT

Coulda, shoulda, woulda. The words of regret that I have found myself saying for the times I didn't follow through on my commitments, especially those commitments that I had more control over. When I have had regrets about my training it has mostly been because I didn't do what I set out to do. It made me feel guilty, and the guilt of not doing the training I had either set out to start, or wanted to continue, made me feel bad about myself.

I have felt at times that I have let myself down and that I only had myself to account to. I have gone through times when I have "excused" my way out of training, whether it was getting out of bed, turning up at my chosen venue to train at, or for my lack of the continuity. The only thing these regrets ended up doing was make it more difficult to get back into it.

Guilt can be a huge demotivator. As human beings we don't always need to be "jazzed up" to go and perform some physical activity, but we want to at least feel a sense of psychological self-esteem, and we like to be in good spirits when it comes to taking up challenges. As humans, we all may often carry some measure of guilt with us, whether it has to do with our relationships, our place in life or the ways we have observed self-care, and as an emotion it can take a wrecking ball to our intentions and motivations toward fitness. So how do you get through the guilt in order to avoid motivational setbacks? I believe the answer is that you simply do not try. Wait, what? Did you just hear that right? "Don't try to get through the guilt?" Some might say or even argue that guilt is essential for self-accountability, and where that may work for highly motivated individuals, I am not here for just them. This book is intended for Joe or Josephine Average and I count myself in this category.

Simply put, the superstars have their internal drive and professional goals for exercising, and if I am being perfectly honest, there are more Joes and Josephines out there who may want to throw a few bucks at the radical set of ideas I have in this book or to use some of the more affordable (free) insights and tools on my website www.justmotivateme.org where I like to share and compare with the community!

So where does the guilt come from? Many things stimulate the feelings of guilt associated with pursuing physical fitness, and here are the ones I have experienced the most through various stages of my own life.

1. You may feel guilty about taking time for yourself when people depend on you, the "indispensability complex." An interesting way to think through this for yourself, is to consider this: If you don't keep in shape, you may be too unfit or incapacitated to be there for people who depend on you.

2. You may experience self-disappointment when you miss or skip a workout for any reason. I think of this as the "beat myself up" complex. This type of guilt complex is usually the most devastating. Setting your own expectations too high can be increasingly self-defeating. I have also noticed that the guilt builds and draws me into a *cycle* of guilt that can hard to break free from.

3. You may feel guilt over how you feel about yourself at the start. The "why even bother" complex can become overwhelming and under-motivating. Guilt can be a very powerful force and is one of the most self-destructive emotions that will appear and do a lot of damage in preventing progress in your journey. What you need to do is to first understand it, then apply a mental circuit breaker that essentially, is you *allowing* yourself to set the guilt to the side to free yourself to reclaim dedication to your fitness routine.

4. I have sometimes felt guilty for lowering my reps or exercise intensity. Don't worry if the reps are not as high or the distance you run.

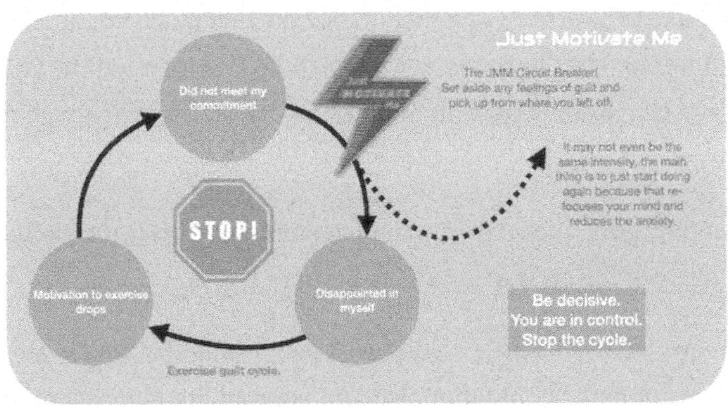

The Guilt Cycle

Accept the skipped workouts and focus on the overall journey. Think more in terms of lifestyle change than singular training efforts and re-focus to accept your skipped workout as something to work on internally. If you find that you cringe at the idea of doing thirty minutes, then commit yourself to asking what you could manage that is less "cringeworthy." You might just find other activities or times that may be more appealing to do something instead of nothing. Once you get back into doing something, then incrementally build upon it.

5. You may feel guilt for not improving the life of your future self. When you bear the guilt of looking at a disappointing future, remind yourself that it is not too late to commit or recommit. I think of this as the "time and tide" complex. There is a saying: "Time and tide wait for no man." Next day, next week, next month, next year will be here before you know it. Live more actively in the present so you can live more effortlessly in the future. Instead of dwelling on guilt or trying to rid yourself of whatever form of guilt may be plaguing your motivation to exercise, accept the guilt for what it actually is and move forward.

As I said earlier, we all carry some sort of guilt—regret that we didn't accomplish something, that we may have not been as good a friend as we would like to have been to someone, or even that we do not do the dishes. If we allow ourselves to become overwhelmed and focus on the guilt, it may become increasingly difficult to make the mental breakthrough necessary to just get on with it.

Accept the guilt, move forward and get moving. This is the circuit breaker that cuts out the cycle of guilt. Believe in it. Use it.

Then give yourself a little credit for at least doing that much. Slowly, your thoughts of guilt should diminish and your ability to develop motivation and *become* motivated, will return in its place. Everyone is very different in this respect, so treat yourself with a little humility and respect and your body will thank you.

CALL TO ACTION

Consider some things through self-reflection about the things that have caused you to feel guilty about your approach to exercise or your experiences in maintaining physical activities in the past.

Have you found yourself being encumbered with the “indispensability complex?” That feeling that you should not do exercise when there are kids to feed or elderly relatives to tend to? Think through the way you use your time and see if you can find a few minutes here and there for exercise. Even little things that are expanded over time, will help.

Do you every experience the “beat myself complex?” If you do, set aside the guilt, tap that mental circuit breaker to stop the guilt cycle and continue.

Have you been troubled by the “why even bother complex?” You are the person who you need to listen to, not all of the perceptions and inner feelings that people may have influenced in the way you feel about yourself. Start something new and work at it on *your* own terms, for you.

In your personal motivation journal, write some brief narratives about the times you felt guilt in not beginning exercise or sticking with it. After that, write an assertion and commitment to yourself in the future. Your future self will be waiting to see how you did. In your own words describe how you will tackle feelings of guilt and why you will tackle them in the way you choose.

"Short cuts make long delays."

J. R. R. Tolkien, The Fellowship of the Ring

17

SHORTCUTS ARE NOT THE WAY

When my kids were little, I tried to instill a sense of "making an effort" as part of teaching them personal responsibility. One of my main mantras was "No shortcuts." If you want to do something properly, make the *effort* and do it *right*. Many people are used to doing the bare minimum to the point of maximum procrastination before the actual "doing" begins.

Not far off the time when the kids were still toddlers, I had written a submission to the Australian Senate, which had called for papers from the experiences of Australian expatriates around the world. I remember writing that among my puzzling observations within the USA was this all-consuming desire for buying more and more stuff and immediate gratification. It gave me pause and made me realize that a significant trait I have observed about society in the USA. Many people really believe you can shortcut so many things in so many ways to achieve your desires.

Ironically, physical effort was actually made when it came to things like the newest smartphone, when people would camp outside their favorite Apple store to satisfy their immediate gratification. When I see the plethora of nutritional supplements for fitness, as well as the equipment you can buy, the DVD and streaming video content and the gym memberships you can subscribe to, it makes my head spin. Most are issued with two things in common: the implied visuals in advertising that the new gadget or training videos will have you looking like a rock star with very little effort, and the disclaimer that results may vary and always consult with your physician first. It is interesting that when I see so many advertised gadgets and gimmicks for fitness being advertised, there is no acknowledgement that every person's motivation to carry out and use products will vary incredibly from person to person. I guess that marketing isn't designed to account for such things.

The bottom line that sank in for me was this. It seemed to me that people have such a strong desire to become more fit and healthy looking that they will believe just about any crap a well-delivered and televised or online marketing campaign will put in front of them, with the implication that things will change their bodies very quickly and with little effort. No shortcuts!

Mentally or physically.

Your mind may be used to finding easy and quick solutions. Don't worry; that happens to the best of us and to most of us. Consider the influences that cause us to think like this. That fancy new fitness machine on TV.

Have you considered the effort you need to make and the time you need to reserve to use it? The new cool gym everyone talks about.

Do you believe you will drag yourself over to the establishment, find parking, change, have the patience to wait on people using equipment that you need to use and even have the self-discipline and knowledge to maintain workouts?

What about if people do not spray, clean and wipe down the big sweat stain they just left on the workout bench you have been waiting for twenty minutes to use because on their rest-breaks they were checking social media for five minutes at a time.

Yes, I have actually witnessed this in real life a LOT. Shortcuts. Ugh! What about the new wonder pill to make you look awesome and fit. Do you really want to believe in the new drug short cut so much? Do you choose to be completely oblivious to the potential side effects, even when the new drug is "natural"?

Commitment actually takes the *will* to win. It takes the understanding about yourself that will set you on the path to making a real difference. You will struggle with having that will if you do not establish and create your very own motivation. For the majority of us *average* folks, you don't just "decide" you have the will to win, nor can you buy it. You need to look within yourself and determine what it is about you specifically, that creates and sustains that powerhouse *will to win* and *keep* winning.

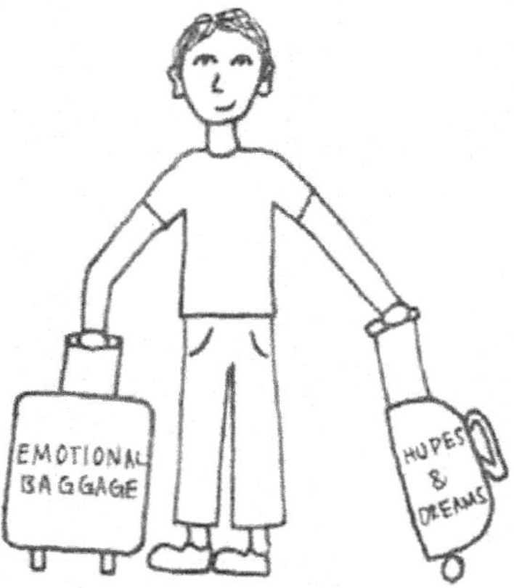

My personal anxieties.

Accept that exercise is an investment in your future health. To do this, you need to believe, not in a supreme being, but in something that makes total sense to you and cannot be denied, at least in your own mind. Try to imagine what "future you" would have wished "current you" had done while trying to manage pain and physical limitations. Accept that even small steps are achievable at the start and that health is a journey, not a destination like losing twenty pounds. Now, getting back to those stimulating marketing campaigns for exercise equipment and gym memberships, I thought of a cheeky little one of my own. It would be grounded in something like this:

You see that gym membership card and remember how much it cost you.

It guilts you.

You see the exercise bike taking space in your bedroom, draped in clothes.

It taunts you.

You see the way your clothes no longer fit like they used to.

It horrifies you.

You experience the loss of things you can no longer seem to do at your age.

It terrifies you.

Shortcuts may feel uplifting but they are short lived and difficult to sustain for a truly motivated fitness journey.

CALL TO ACTION

Consider the things that you may be drawn to as shortcuts. In your personal motivation journal, write down the marketed services or products or even circumstances that are *your* shortcuts.

Write down a personal attestation on how you feel about these shortcuts, whether they are real or perceived, and how you intend to deal with them in the future.

Imagine yourself in the future, disappointed in how your body has coped with age, and write down a message that your future self may have wanted you to hear in the present. As your future self, what would you think you could tell your present self to work on more?

Consider how much better you would feel about yourself in the future if you realized you had at least made an effort!

If you have a list of things you have invested in over the years, you may want to inventory them and the approximate money you spent on it all.

Now, consider how helpful it all was and re-focus on less spending on stuff – at least for now. Train your mind to train your body, and remember there are a lot of things that you can do for free! Walking, stretching, finding small weights around the house, and even doing chores or clearing away that clutter that has plagued you for so long.

Making physical efforts to do essential life management tasks can help your life in general and also burn a few calories so why would you *not* want to do it?

You may find out, as I have with myself, that you can get into a "mode" and just keep going and feel good about what you accomplish when you choose *not* to take the short cut.

"To be yourself in a world that is constantly trying to make you something else is the greatest accomplishment."

Ralph Waldo Emerson

18

HOW DO WE DEFINE OUR ACCOMPLISHMENTS?

It was December 2014 in a very cold Ohio. I remember that I was in that stage of martial arts training where I was about to test for first-degree black belt in martial arts. As a fifty-year-old, I was most likely ready for the final test that would consist of techniques in sequence, sparring, self-defense, board breaking, and general knowledge and attitude. It would test my mastery of what I had learned in my journey to black belt rank. I remember feeling pretty nervous about taking the test and wanting to first reassure myself of my own abilities in order to boost my confidence.

During the Christmas week, the temperatures were very low. I picked a day to do some outdoor training. It was minus five degrees Fahrenheit or minus twenty degrees Celsius (for non-Americans), and I decided on this particular day to train by our very own local "Hoover Dam." Not *THE* Hoover Dam, I think this smaller dam might have been named after the vacuum cleaner and not the President. I packed my things and drove over. I had a beanie, a jacket, gloves and a thirty-pound weight vest. The stairs that ascended each side of the dam were 104 in number, and for thirty minutes, with my face freezing, I went up and down those stairs wearing my weight vest breathing cold air and warming up my body with the exertion. I did have company that day, though. The only other person out there was a Marine in training, wearing a backpack doing the same thing on the stairs on the other side of the dam. This experience taught me that if I was to overcome obstacles, I had to make a determined effort to go the extra mile to reap the rewards at the end. Of course, this level of physical training was totally unnecessary for the demands of my testing but what I was actually doing was training my mind to achieve a sense of discipline, confidence in myself and to gain a feeling of accomplishment. Training the mind can also be done *through* training the body it seems. I have come to understand that training the mind and training the body may be a concept very much like the yin yang symbol. Even within the mind there is the yin/yang notion of the left brain / right brain – the ways in which your brain works to focus and analyze on mechanics and tasks while at the same time looking at the broader picture and longer-term view. Yin and Yang. Opposites, yet interlocked and in balance with each other.

We often talk among our friends and family about the things that we feel proud of, especially as we do the things that are difficult. We are often conditioned to expect what people usually talk about when they associate accomplishments in the realm of personal health and physical appearance. In many typical Western social circles, it is common to hear commentary about the amount of weight someone lost, the number of dress sizes someone went down, how much weight someone was able to bench press in the gym or how far someone was able to continuously run or jog.

While these may all be significant accomplishments, they all usually share one defining characteristic: they are achieved at a specific point in time. People fail to realize that these accomplishments are in fact, the pinnacle but not the true accomplishment itself. The true accomplishments, I feel, are the positive results made apparent in your life from your physical accomplishments. Having more energy to play with his kids would be a great accomplishment for a father who wants a great relationship with his children. Lowering cholesterol means your family no longer needs to worry as much about hypertension-related illnesses or cardiac events. Landing that movie role or passing your military recruit course are other life-changing accomplishments.

When I was halfway through the colored belts in my journey to a first-degree black belt, I remember telling people that the incremental achievements in belt rank, as important as they were to me, were not replaced by an ever-greater aspiration to change my lifestyle in ways that altered my mental age as well as my physical capabilities. I also went on to further and evolve my motivations for helping others through becoming a black belt and then to become a certified instructor myself. I think it is great to also recognize and celebrate accomplishments of your personal growth.

How much have you learned about nutrition, biomechanics, anatomy, your own journey of developing self-discipline? These things individually or collectively are incredible accomplishments. Accomplishments can and should be so much more than the arbitrary things that are most common to most people. Accomplishments are *food* for *future* reflection to shape or even restore motivation and are important to you, personally. They are the things that matter in terms of your quality of life and lifestyle. Sometimes, your own personal accomplishments may indirectly and positively improve the lifestyle of family and friends.

CALL TO ACTION

What achievements in your life, big or small, have provided a sense of accomplishment? What have you seen in others that inspired you?

For some, having children, finding their dream job or achieving an academic goal, provided a feeling of accomplishment. For the things you had to work at, think about the inner motivations at play during that time, and how you went about applying that motivation to your end goals.

When you think about it, there is usually something you did for yourself, or something you did or sacrificed for others. It is something that improved an outcome in a person's life whether it was yours or someone else's.

Write these reflections in your personal motivation journal so you can refer to them in the future to reinforce and remind yourself of how your accomplishments of the past were linked to some intrinsic motivations you were experiencing at that time.

Now, imagine some of the lifestyle accomplishments you can drive towards *today* and see if these are the things your future self would like to reflect upon with positivity and less regrets. These maybe things like sustained exercise workouts, daily walks, regular stretches. Small or large, accomplishments are all important. Write these things down too. You may think of them as near-term goals that you want to count for something that your future self will appreciate.

"Our very survival depends on our ability to stay awake, to adjust to new ideas, to remain vigilant and to face the challenge of change."

Martin Luther King Jr.

19

WHAT DRIVES MOTIVATION?

Many times throughout history, people have undertaken great and difficult things with tremendous motivation. In 1973, Apollo Thirteen was on its way to the moon, and during that journey, the NASA flight control center heard those alarming words: "Houston, we have a problem." After analysis and verification, it rapidly became apparent that not only was the mission to the moon at risk, but also, the lives of the Apollo astronauts who were now traveling in a damaged spacecraft that was venting oxygen. The story went beyond NASA and the USA and in fact, traveled the entire world.

It could be said that the original message from the astronauts triggered the initial motivation to do something difficult. To respond to a crisis where lives hung in the balance. Later during this event, flight control director Gene Krantz steered his leadership toward responding to this crisis swiftly and was quoted as saying, "Failure is not an option." Within this context and given the urgency of the situation, this motivated all the ground crew experts, in co-ordination with experienced astronauts and scientists to work around the clock in analysis, simulations and innovations to ensure that the astronauts could be helped remotely, while their spacecraft was outside of the earth's orbit. Maintaining motivation was the order of the day, to keep going, no matter what.

As history reminds us, the dedication of so many highly motivated people surprised the world in a rescue and recovery operation that to this day is still seen as one of NASA's greatest success stories.

Many things can drive motivation. Some may inspire you, while some might make you feel good and some may drive logic and reasoning. It may be inspiring to you when you see people who are older in age than you, who tend to look and act with a much more youthful exuberance. It may be encouraging to see how much more effortlessly certain people may tackle physical actions and give you hope for the types of things you may want to strive for.

Things that may make you feel good include experiencing certain wins or "bragging rights" that you earned after training for many months to successfully run your first marathon. It may even be the "runner's high" or release of endorphins that occurs in the brain after a particularly difficult physical challenge.

Often, along with feeling good, you may also want to like the way you look. It might be to be more toned or to look better in the way clothes fit you. It is a very common motivation.

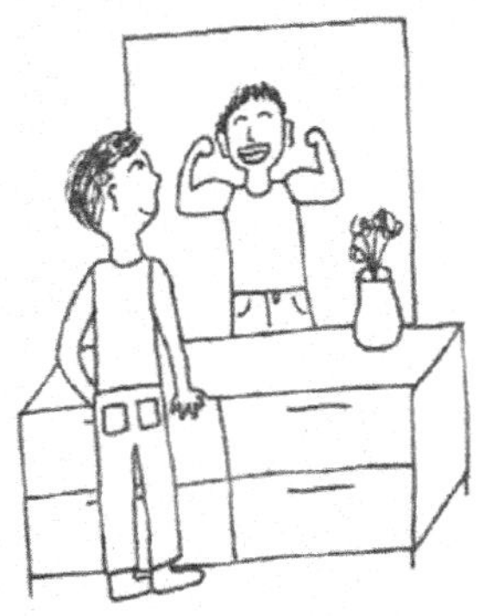

What I imagine in my future self.

Things that are driven by logic or reasoning may include factors such as your ability to tackle challenges, improve your health, make love for much longer or even develop more focus and clarity toward your work. Whatever drives motivation, remember that motivation is always personal. This is because everyone's backstory and life experiences differ.

Consider these possibilities that may shape or drive yourself:

I am *obligated* to get in shape because the military branch I belong to, demands it.

I am *compelled* to lose weight so I will look good on my wedding day.

I *want* to exercise because I know a healthy body boosts my immunity and brain health.

I *need* to become healthy or I won't live to see my next birthday.

Ask yourself what factors or circumstances represent motivations, and, better yet, also ask your friends and family what *they* believe motivates you. You might be surprised by their answers, but this is because their window into your life is from an entirely different perspective.

CALL TO ACTION

What have you learned about yourself or some of the people closest to you that drives or inspires motivation to do difficult things?

Motivation is indeed very personal and related to different times in each person's life. For example, the motivation to study for a tertiary academic award such as a diploma or a degree might be to land a better job that will lead to a promising career.

The motivation to train hard physically and mentally might be essential for someone to pursue their dream of becoming a dancer for a prestigious ballet company. It may also be to develop a mastery of a certain style of ancient self-defense or fighting techniques.

While performing arts or martial arts may be compelling for some people, for others, it may be the desire to be able to partake in certain activities that are quite simple and still fun.

When you discover what inspires and motivates you to do challenging or even simpler things, take a moment to consider those things and make updates to your personal motivation journal.

You may have also observed behaviors in others or even throughout history that connect with you. Summarize these as well.

"I suppose it is tempting, if the only tool you have is a hammer, to treat everything as if it were a nail."

DR. ABRAHAM H. MASLOW.

20

WHAT YOU NEED

Back in 1997, I was preparing to leave my lifelong home of Australia to emigrate to the United States. It was a tough move and definitely a landmark decision that would affect my life for many years to come. When I lived in Australia, I knew of many immigrants from places all over the world. Some came as refugees with very little and some came as part of sponsored programs in the British Commonwealth of Nations to live and contribute to the prosperity of Australia. I never really considered what these people had moved away from and what their new needs and desires would be. So, as I was planning *my* move, it got me to thinking about what I wanted to take with me, but more importantly, what I *needed* to take with me. After all, how hard could it be?

I made list after list of the things I thought I would need for basic living, identification, finding work, establishing myself as a resident alien and making sure I could adapt to the new health care system. After careful introspection, research and strategic thinking, I arrived at the set of items that would meet most if not all of my most immediate needs. I learned a lot from this experience. I learned about the things that gave me happiness, made me feel secure and supported me in day-to-day living. I also learned a lot about the things that I could do or get by without. I found that understanding my deepest needs made me more knowledgeable about future personal growth. *Applying* this knowledge would help me create the motivation necessary for my numerous life changes over the next few years.

Marriage, finding work, having kids, obtaining US citizenship, purchasing a home and all of the new professional and personal adjustments, including health, revealed many new needs for my life in America.

When you begin to understand how you can relate your own needs to your motivations, these motivations can become very powerful in elevating you to building a better version of yourself. Those motivations have served me for many years. If motivation is at the center of equipping ourselves with focus, determination and learning toward training, then our innate hierarchy of personal needs is at the center of our motivation. In the early twentieth century, a famous psychologist, Dr. Maslow, determined that human beings act within a basic framework of evolving needs that are met through the choices, actions and circumstances that surround us from the time we are born.

Our needs stem from physiological factors that act as our basic life support like oxygen, food, water, shelter and climate all the way through safety needs, sense of love and belonging, self-esteem and accomplishment to self-actualization. Understanding our needs is essential to understanding ourselves, and understanding ourselves is essential to knowing what motivates us, why it motivates us and how lasting the motivation can be. We may find that we are motivated to do big things through pure grit and self-determination but that our ability to sustain is limited. We may also find that we can overcome physical challenges and train ourselves to be highly active in physical pursuits if it means that our kids get dinner on the table every night. In all of this, everyone is different. This is why I believe that sometimes and indeed, many times, when people buy into a gym membership or a fitness group or purchase a yoga mat, their tendency is to allow their physical training to deteriorate over time.

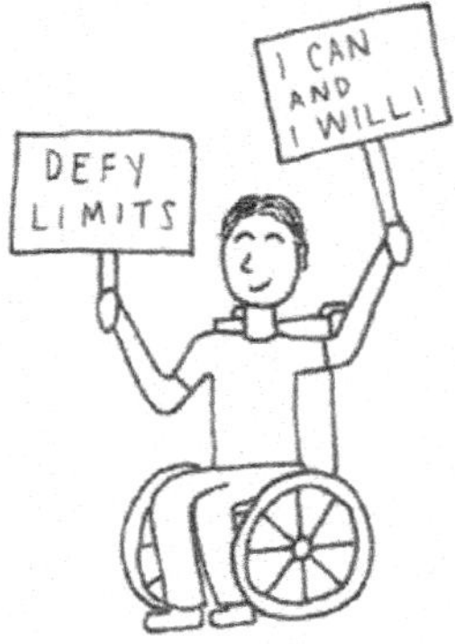

Overcoming challenges.

People are different based upon many factors such as socioeconomic circumstances, physical characteristics, mental health characteristics, personal responsibilities, life experiences and many other things. I love to use Maslow's hierarchy of needs as a framework for personal introspection into what I really *need* in life. It may only be what I *think* I need, but we have to start somewhere right?

Training for your current self and for your future self.

When I look at the needs that align with motivation for physical training, I see the needs in two levels. The first level of needs is focused on personal training for the here and now and mostly rests with self-esteem and belonging. The necessity to train is directly connected to my desire to feel good about my ability to pursue fun activities like skiing, mountaineering and hiking as well as my desire to learn and accomplish different techniques and levels of mastery in martial arts.

The second level of needs is focused on personal training for my future self. As someone who has always been a strategic thinker, I often consider, just short of the point of obsession, the expectations I have of my future self. I regard my future self as post retirement and into senior age living and as connected more into physiological and safety needs. I cannot bear the thought of being debilitated later in life and then reflecting upon my younger days and thinking, *Why the bloody hell didn't you work on your fitness THEN? Look at yourself now, you are always in pain, everything is a monumental effort and you are putting an unnecessary strain on your loved ones.* I keep these two levels in mind before, during and after training, and they serve as strong motivators based on my current needs as well as my future needs.

CALL TO ACTION

Needs are very personal. We all have different needs, and we are affected by just about everything that surrounds us in our day-to-day circumstances. Our needs change with the passage of time, and this reminds me of the things I have been used to people telling me in conversations throughout my own life.

Here are some typical examples:

"You don't really understand, just wait until you get married."

So, then I get married and then all I hear is this:

"Really? Just wait until you have kids!"

So, then I have kids and then I begin to hear more of this:

"That may be so, but you won't really know what it's like until you're on a fixed income."

It is at this point that I usually head to that place that is further from the crankiness and closer to the alcohol.

Yes, my needs have evolved and many were difficult to predict, well, maybe except the ones at the bottom of Maslow's hierarchy of needs—physiological and safety needs. In your personal motivation journal, write down three reasons to pursue fitness that would satisfy your physiological needs and three more reasons to work on your fitness to address your safety needs.

Here are some examples to get you thinking:

Physiological: *I need to become fit so that I have higher resistance to colds, improved connective tissue and stronger bones.*

Safety: *I need to become fit so that I can make my way up and down stairs with little to no risk of collapsing from exhaustion or poor joint health.*

"The best time to plant a tree was twenty years ago. The second-best time is now."

CHINESE PROVERB

21

SHORT-TERM MOTIVATION

I have developed short-term motivation many times, through various life experiences, and I learned that you get to the point where you do actually recognize it when you see it, whether in yourself or in others. It is not a bad thing. In fact, short-term motivation is that excitement that people feel when they have something to feel good about doing. Seeing an infomercial on body sculpting devices or fitness programs with enticing deals makes the deal seem like a win-win. You get to have the "look" you crave *and* for half the cost!

Many years ago, my daughter Cassie was involved in dance and the dance studio put on a yearly event called the "Father Daughter Ballet". This was a chance for a handful of superb specimens of dad-bods to train in ballet with their respective daughters. The commitment for this was about ten weeks and at the end, we would all participate at the big recital, tutus and all. That's the daughters, not the dads! So, it was a short term and I was motivated. Training my mind for this was easy. I wanted to create a special memory with my daughter and do something fun at the same time. Cassie and I did very well, in fact we did it two years in a row and have a couple of nice trophies. I learned one thing apart from ballet though. While I was doing the father-daughter ballet, I was also practicing martial arts on other nights. What I came to realize was that the ballet training was much harder!

Today, I train hard four days a week in my basement gym, and I mix cardio with stretches, planks and a mixed workout of five hundred reps for core, strength and flexibility. I train harder and more consistently than I did during my soldiering years, and I am lathered in sweat at the end of each workout. I have proven to myself that short-term motivation can be very effective when you know the *importance* of what you are setting out to accomplish. I have also learned that it is never too late to pick things up again. What gets us motivated in the short term? I have often heard of people wanting to shed a few pounds to fit into their favorite clothes, to fulfill a New Year resolution to work off those Thanksgiving or Christmas dinners, or to get their "beach-bod" on in readiness for the summer.

Short-term motivation can be great for deciding to begin a journey, but more often than not, those reasons for short-term motivation will not work for sustaining a routine of exercise and general fitness. When the wedding is over, we hang up the dress or the tux and then relax. We relax our attitudes where it concerns diet and exercise. Exercise is the easier one to ignore, whereas diet presents a constant and visual reminder of what and how much you choose to put into your body. It is important therefore, not to confuse the things that give you short-term motivation with the things you believe will keep you fit and active. Short-term motivation is driven by the information that is most easily available and consumed by the masses. People want information to be simple and the imagery to be stimulating in ways that make sense.

Buy a stability ball or a jump rope in some fancy packaging and chances are there will be a small booklet or picture chart of the types of exercise you can do to whip your body into shape. Scores of fitness books describe the mechanics of how to "get fit." Surely these are valuable in ways that help people to learn techniques to improve fitness. If you need to learn how to improve your endurance, your strength, your flexibility or your waistline, then traditional literature is there for the taking.

We are not all athletes or superstars.

For *some* people, this literature will really work for its intended purpose, for *some* of the time. For some people, after purchases are made, they will end up hardly noticed or read, and it will find a final resting place with several other purchases that seemed like a good idea at the time.

This is why many people have well-cluttered basements, storage facilities and garages. I am a little embarrassed to say this, but I am real example of this. My gym has a punching bag that went unused for almost twenty years until I really began to use it. Same goes for many other pieces of equipment that I own and have now seen more service in the past four years than in the past twenty. Training my mind in order to train my body made all the difference. Try to use things that you learn about yourself and not the information that comes in a wrapper. What you learn about yourself is that you can develop and drive short-term, achievable objectives and gradually turn them into long-term habits.

For example, if you ask yourself why you may not look good in that tuxedo, examine the circumstances that led you to that conclusion. If the real root cause is that you carry too much weight as your "norm," then maybe you want to find a new "norm." Using your mind, you may teach yourself that you want to accomplish a long-term goal that will help you meet many objectives all of the time. The dedication to a one-month effort can sometimes make a big difference towards establishing a routine. I have found this true for myself and it has worked for me.

Allow yourself to do less than you're capable of at the start.

The thing to remember is that for a habit of activity, you should accept that it is quite reasonable and ok to begin slowly at the very start, even doing less than you're probably capable of. Why do less than you're capable of? Surely no fitness advisor would say such a thing? Luckily, I am not a fitness advisor. I am someone who is imparting some insights and learnings that happened to work through experimentation, error and adaptation. I learned that even though I could sometimes do way more, as governed by my natural drive and personality, the body *was* getting trained but the mind was not being trained to the more lasting habit of a fitness routine. You need to be gentle on yourself and grow into it. Being gentle on yourself means being gentle on yourself mentally—don't feel guilty for doing so little at the start—and also be gentle on yourself physically. If a minute is all you can do, then do a minute and give yourself a little credit. Something small, will still help you train your mind, while the alternative, doing nothing, trains well, nothing.

CALL TO ACTION

Explore your memories or observations of others where you have seen short-term motivations at work. For your personal memories, think about the allure at the time that motivated you toward becoming fitness oriented to the point that inspired you to take action.

Now consider how long that motivation lasted and try to remember what you did after.

Did you build upon your motivation to make yourself fitness oriented in the long term?

If you did, was it the same motivation source you began with or something different?

If your short-term motivation accomplished some goal, did you ever think of what it would be like to keep training?

If not, what held you back? Lack of interest? Feeling like you wanted to do just the bare minimum?

Do you wish you had done something differently, or were you happy with the way things turned out then? Now?

Think about how you might feel to try a new routine for a month, where your first workouts are significantly shorter or less intensive than what you are capable of at the start, with a gradual increase over the weeks.

With these observations, I encourage you to write down your discoveries in your personal motivation journal.

"Physical fitness is not only one of the most important keys to a healthy body, it is the basis of dynamic and creative intellectual activity."

John F. Kennedy

22

LONG-TERM MOTIVATION

I remember back in the year 1982 when I was taking math in my senior year of high school. We had to study a unit about the fundamentals of computing. I had never seen a computer system up close, save for the home computers that my friends had, mainly for playing computer games on. Other than that, all of my familiarity with computers came from what I had seen in sci-fi movies. During this final unit in our mathematics curriculum, I was exposed to the ways in which computers work to process information. The closest I had come to this in the past was creating letters on a typewriter. How could I ever have guessed that the world of computers would create a long-term motivation to pursue knowledge, so much so that it actually launched my career?

On reflection, many factors influenced my motivation as an eighteen-year-old, my motivations always adjusting as my life situations and circumstances evolved over the years. Some of these motivations became long term motivations which still influence me to this day. You see, I believe that the factors that drive long-term motivation for many things may essentially be very similar, no matter what the motivation is really about.

At an early age, I had abundant curiosity and the mindset of an engineer who wanted to create things that were sophisticated, required problem-solving skills and were always open to change. As my years advanced, I still claimed the same motivations as when I was younger, but I introduced new motivations such as how I defined myself professionally, the effect of how my work was used in commercial applications and the money I could make when I delved deeper into the ever-changing and evolving field of information systems.

At the center of all of these things are my personal needs. Every human possesses needs, no matter their ethnicity, social status, background, religious beliefs, political affiliations, education or gender. Over time, we master our understanding of what our needs are, as we go through every stage of life and even as we begin to fulfill our needs along the way.

JFK was a big picture thinker.

It is interesting to understand how our needs are crucial to motivation in the short-term and long-term aspects of our endeavors. What I love about JFK's quote cited at the beginning of this chapter, is that it is a remarkable example of big-picture thinking. JFK was right in believing and promoting the linkage of a healthy body to the basis of dynamic and creative activity. Keeping healthy improves your mental health and ability to think clearly. Furthermore, distractions such as illness can be lowered, as your fitness helps you build a tougher immune system.

Being more active helps to pump more blood and fresh oxygen throughout the body, including the brain, to support a healthier mind for thinking and coping with life's challenges. Imagine creating new neurons! Yes, neuroplasticity is a fascinating area of medical science. The ability to see changes in the brain, such as the formation of brand-new neurons (brain cells) through exercise.

A healthy brain is one of my personal strongest motivators to keep exercising, and in many of the Eastern doctrines and concepts like yin and yang, mind and body will always have a strong and even symbiotic relationship, so keep them both strong. You might consider that we use beliefs, behaviors or other drivers for strategic motivation and they surround us all in everyday life.

We seem more willing to commit to completing a university degree or to put away some money regularly for retirement planning. So why do we still falter when it comes to motivating ourselves in fitness? In the previous chapter, we discussed short-term motivation that may take you to the edge of habit forming—usually after a month of continual commitment and focus. A month can fly by, but many things can break habits, and these are the excuses we make for ourselves. Have you ever noticed that whenever you are trying to argue with yourself, you always win? That's true, but then you also lose.

As you start your journey, see what helps you with physical activity and what robs your motivation. For example, if music gets you pumped up, then play your music! If doing repetitive styles of exercise begins to feel like you're on a hamster-wheel, then change it up and introduce some variety.

Variety is also good in exercise because it helps to activate different muscle groups at varying intervals while allowing other muscle groups to recover. If you can last a month, do something special for yourself or for your friend, loved one or colleague for whom your encouragement and celebration will count. Now, further down the track, if you can take it to six months, then you have a better chance at incorporating your journey as part of your lifestyle.

I realized that with martial arts, I began to see surprising and positive changes for my health after the first month, but it wasn't until about just under a year that I began to feel that this activity needed to become part of my lifestyle. I have practiced martial arts for more than eight years, which is the longest I have been able to continuously maintain an activity in my life.

"What's in it for me" and "immediate gratification" are two powerful drivers that lead people to be motivated to do certain things, but what are the other drivers? Could it be something like "out of sight out of mind"? Perhaps if we don't "see" the retirement funds coming out, we just get used to the disposable income that remains in our paycheck. If we see a month over month improvement in energy, strength or flexibility, does this help to maintain an interest in martial arts? Sometimes, benefits are not so obvious until you acknowledge them and at that point, it is a good time to reflect upon understanding the things you did to bring about those benefits.

CALL TO ACTION

Take a look at something about your life, and I really mean for the *majority* of your life, that you feel has always been positive and something that you succeeded at that has been unwavering.

Maybe you have always enjoyed gardening or loved playing music or had a passion for helping people.

Now reflect on your motivations during the fulfillment of this activity and how your motivations may have remained the same or even adjusted over time, while maintaining your overall motivation.

The final step is to *just write it* down. Your personal motivation journal is just the place to do this. Keep it for reference and build upon it as you continue your voyage of constant self-rediscovery that will help you motivate yourself toward being a more fit version of yourself.

Bonus Chapter 1

THE POWER OF THE MIND-BODY CONNECTION

Motivation starts with your mind, and your brain is the physical powerhouse that allows your mind to operate. The mind and body connection is not just some mystical thing we hear about from eastern philosophies. It is fundamental to how we, as humans operate as whole beings. The importance of this connection is something I have come to learn and appreciate only in later years of life, and along the way, science has shown evidence of how this connection manifests in ways that are awesome to witness.

Brain science is becoming more and more significant in showing us the way the mind works and its relationship to our whole selves. If we exercise more, we can reduce stress and improve our immune system. Furthermore, more blood flow to the brain can help to develop more physical brain! Certain neurochemistry triggers and actions will interplay with feelings of mood, happiness, drive, accomplishment and persistence, and a basic summary of these is provided below. This summary is not offered as medical expertise or advice. However, we can begin to witness and learn from the mind-body connection through exercise. Now, if we explore what we witness even further, we can use this knowledge to grow and stimulate our *personal* motivation for exercise.

The mind-body connection is an important aspect of our health and wellness that we should never undervalue or trivialize. I have learned of its existence, its value and its importance in all of the physical training endeavors I have undertaken. It is also the connection that we *need* to learn more about in ourselves as we train the mind to train the body.

I have understood things about my mind-body connection that have enabled me to realize that there are different aspects of physical training intensity to acknowledge and I have constructed these below.

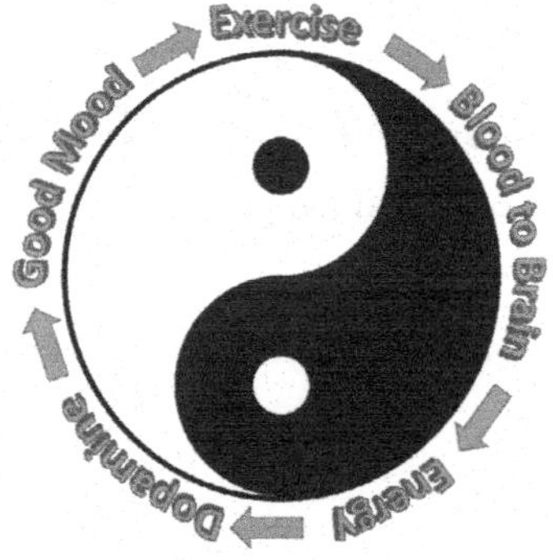

Low intensity workout cycle.

A low intensity workout is definitely the place to start. These can be somewhere in the range of say 30 seconds to a few minutes. These workouts are excellent to train your mind into the *routine* of doing activity, while beginning a very light workout for your body. There is a cycle here. Do a little exercise, increase the blood flow to the brain. Start to see the way you're your mind begins to think more clearly and your body begins to have more energy. This affects your mood to boost your motivation to do what? More exercise! Just don't overdo it. Keep it simple, increase gradually but steadily.

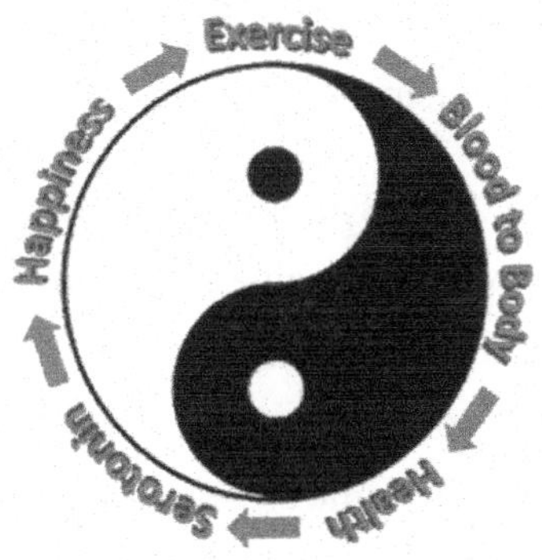
Exercise
Blood to Body
Health
Serotonin
Happiness

Medium intensity workout cycle.

A medium intensity workout last about 10 minutes to around 30 minutes. It is the type of workout where you could do a little variety of cardio, maybe some core and strength. Again, there is a cycle that involves the effects of physical activity on blood flow, healthier body and mood. Many personal trainers will offer a 30-minute workout option and these types of workouts are ideal if you have time during a midday break during your work schedule, or early in the morning. It is the perfect workout to use as a way of maintaining general fitness, but always strive to change it up from time to time.

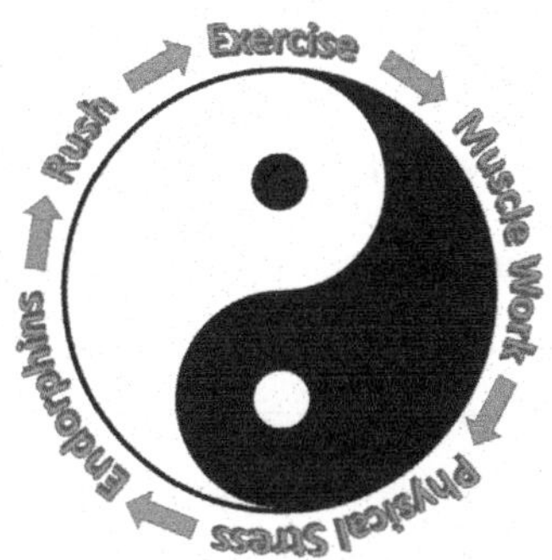
Exercise
Muscle Work
Physical Stress
Endorphins
Rush

High intensity workout cycle.

A high intensity workout is usually one that takes more than 30 minutes and may last for a few hours. This may be an event like a exercise class, or a half marathon that you participate in, it may also be a whole afternoon of rappelling and rock climbing. High intensity may also be less time but more speed and quicker transitions in the regular training you do. I have seen people taking rest breaks during workouts in gyms, to just look up at the TV screens and watch the news for about 10 minutes in their 30minute workout. Not that intense, except in the way it is posted in their social media! You will know for *yourself* when your workout is intense.

It is satisfying to know that your body can produce chemical neurotransmitters that are all part of the mind-body connection. This is nothing new. The mind and the body have a very special connection, and my choice of the yin/yang connection was very deliberate.

Ancient medicines and philosophies have known this for thousands of years, but in the West, we mostly treat symbols like this as a cool thing to string around your neck. In martial arts, we treat this symbol with some reverence and as a reminder that all things that may be opposing forces, may also work together in balance and harmony.

If our mind blocks our motivation to work out, our body suffers. But if the mind can be trained to accept the value of training the body, it can lead to a healthier body, and that satisfaction and energy can lead to a healthier mind that is more accepting of the training and its evolution from small steps to habit to lifestyle. The appropriate resource for medical advice will always be medical professionals, but it would help them immensely if you are very open and honest about your concerns, your goals and your feelings so that they may offer advice to promote motivation. Remember that you are different to everyone else, even if you are a twin.

Bonus Chapter 2

FIND YOUR "SETTING"

This bonus chapter is about what can and inevitably does happen from time to time for many people, so let me share my ideas here.

Imagine for a minute that after much introspection and self-study, you have come around to actually motivating yourself to move from the couch to a form of physical exercise. You are excited because you have *reason* and *belief* as two motivational "guides" at your side, bringing you forward to undertake a workout or jog. After a short while, you realize your motivation begins to dip. What's wrong? You definitely are motivated by the benefits you understand, you also have come to know how to focus your attitude in a way that makes sense to you, and yet you are less than thrilled about the impending exercise.

It could be that you need to find the right setting that makes exercise more appealing or even manageable for your personal comfort and enjoyment. Here are ten settings to consider.

Once you have determined your setting *preferences*, use this knowledge to shape the circumstances, environments and tools that will motivate you to do exercise!

These settings will be great to compare against the type of exercise scenarios that are likely to work best. For example, a gym where groups work out together, or a learning exercise like martial arts or even something with a musical backtrack and rhythm like dance.

Setting number 1. Sound.

Do you prefer an atmosphere of energetic sound or quiet? Do you need quiet to focus on your exercise, or do noisy places provide more workout stimulation for you? Maybe it depends.

Setting number 2. Existence.

Do you do better with solitude or with company? Some people prefer the privacy of their space or the intimacy of working with a partner or personal trainer.

Setting number 3. Ambience.

Do you like a bright or dim setting? How do you respond with lighting? Do you like it to be bright and invigorating or dim and easy on the eyes?

Setting number 4. Rhythm.

Do you like to get in your groove with music that raises the pulse or stills the mind? Some people like a steady beat, whether it is classical and soothing or restless and loud like hard rock. Do you have a preference?

Setting number 5. Clothing.

Do you like clothes that are loose and soft or trendy and tight fitting? Working out should be comfortable. There are demands from movement and from perspiration. How do you see yourself in workout gear?

Setting number 6. Environment.

Are you an indoors person or an outdoors person? The weather can always be a factor. But if the weather was favorable, would you prefer indoor or outdoor activity?

Setting number 7. Resistance.

Do you prefer your own body or machines and other resistance devices like weights? Do you feel more motivated to use your own body weight or machines or other devices? Maybe you like to mix it all up.

Setting number 8. Measurement.

Do you prefer to use your gut-feeling or instruments? Do you need to track progress? Maybe its weight, waistline, distance or reps. What works for you? Gadgets or gut feel?

Setting number 9. Place.

Are you happier working out in a more familiar place like home or a fresh place like a gym, community center or park? Is your home where you feel safer to work out? Maybe it's a gym your friends go to, but on some days, there's nothing quite like a park!

Setting number 10. Drive.

Do you prefer competing against yourself or others? What gets you going more? Maybe you like to achieve a bump in self-esteem through beating your personal best. Maybe you like to be in friendly competition with others.

Take the preferences you have determined for yourself in each of the ten categories and write them up in your Personal Motivation Journal.

When considering that next exercise idea, that new exercise class or gym membership, consult what you have learned about yourself in terms of preferences!

Bonus Chapter 3

LESSONS LEARNED FROM BRUCE LEE

Bruce Lee is probably the martial artist for whom I have the deepest admiration. I respect his warrior attitude to all things in life. He was a brave immigrant, a relentless spirit driven to mastery of everything and anything he set his mind to and a devoted husband and father. I loved seeing photos of him with his kids. His legacy is alive and strong today, abundantly available in his teachings, literature and the work of his family.

Bruce Lee embodied the warrior spirit in its most spectacular form and in his powerful attitude toward training. Bruce knew that to be superbly skilled and to achieve mastery in martial arts, he had to put in the effort effectively and constantly. He applied his mind to the task first. Ideas, feelings, planning, vision – all these things that would help him to establish his own work in America.

He would also seek to differentiate his style from that of other "traditional" martial arts schools. Bruce Lee knew that to achieve these goals, he would have to set a much higher expectation of training.

He had various motivational factors, from being fit enough to defend himself from the violence he experienced in the streets of Hong Kong in his earlier years, to having the flexibility and strength required for him to rise to number one in the Hong Kong Cha-Cha dance community and later to become an expert martial artist who would require a strong physique with strength and flexibility, to learning and incorporating techniques and styles from a variety of fighting art forms.

During his career, Bruce Lee undoubtedly had many injury setbacks, the most notable one being the time that he sustained a painful and significant injury after a fight, an injury so severe that doctors speculated that he would never practice martial arts again and may even have difficulties with everyday mobility. Of course, Bruce had already developed a warrior mentality that simply refused to surrender to this injury setback and found the mental strength and determination to fix himself in ways that medical practitioners at the time thought were near to impossible.

On a personal note, I have experienced temporary physical setbacks through injury or illness that through determination and will I have been able to overcome, including injuries to my wrists, hands, back and knees. Having a trained mind helped me overcome these setbacks and continue my fitness journey. Nothing compared to Bruce Lee, but the mindset is something I like to believe we may share.

Bonus Chapter 4

TRAINER INSIGHTS

In order to provide a broader perspective on the motivation for fitness, it was essential to incorporate lessons from people in the field who share the responsibility and passion for bringing out the best in people through fitness training. I chose to avoid trainers who are more involved with professional athletes or sports adventurers because this book needs to address the motivational philosophies and ideas that are relatable and relevant to everyday people.

The trainers I spoke with are all community-based trainers involved with activities that require levels of physical training, self-discipline and persistence. I have also included general insights shared with me through years of martial arts, yoga and friends who have learned to train themselves. The aim was to unearth the aspects of motivation that these trainers observe, drive or work through with their trainees and to reveal behavioral trends and challenges that cross the broad spectrum of activities.

Personal trainers are some of the most motivated people you will ever meet. It was interesting to learn that the things that motivated them to become personal trainers were things like a desire to see change in people, or even having endured the challenges of learning how to train and then understanding the value of helping people with those same challenges.

One trainer said that when she started going to the gym as someone who wanted to get fit, she would look up YouTube videos on how to use exercise equipment and knew that she probably wasn't the only one. The best trainers tend to have a great set of technical skills for exercise and an understanding of body mechanics, but more than anything, they have empathy and enthusiasm.

Meeting people where they are.

The desire to meet people where they are, to acknowledge their challenges and to give them hope is absolutely essential. This is something I learned from my Master instructors in martial arts. I have also seen this with yoga instructors and it is so essential to helping people to develop a mindset that allows them to believe in themselves.

I also learned from trainers that they see a definite change in the mental state of their clients in terms of becoming more positive, having higher self-esteem and a desire to keep going. Finding a good trainer, whether it is for personal fitness, martial arts or yoga, should involve a conversation before signing up. Get to know why they do what they do, and ask them about techniques that they use. Another trainer I spoke with told me that keeping people accountable often involves getting to the root of issues that are at odds with their training discipline.

Understanding the "why" was also a technique that this trainer used and is a fundamental part of understanding how it impacts clients' outlook and willingness to keep training and their ability to sustain it. Like most of us, trainers endure setbacks, and it was interesting to hear how they overcame them. One trainer shared that overcoming setbacks was possible by reminding herself that she overcame challenges in the past and that she could do it again. Another thing was self-accountability to the investment that was made in time and also in buying equipment.

Several trainers remarked on reminding themselves of their sense of duty to people as their trainer and also to be a positive example for their clients. When you think you have found your trainer, make sure that you tell them about any limitations you have, especially any medical conditions, prior surgeries and general activities that require physical effort. Many will do this as part of an initial assessment.

Find *your* why.

I think it helps to let them know your goals and your "why," in other words, why you want to undertake training at all. For martial arts, it may be to gain confidence or to be able to defend yourself; for yoga, it may be to become more flexible and to exercise your body in more gentle and meditative ways. You may also want to join a dance class because you love rhythm and find that the workout is less noticeable when you are immersed in music and movement. For personal training, it may be so that you can take that adventure vacation and not become exhausted hiking through the foothills of the Himalayas.

Bonus Chapter 5

YOUR PERSONAL MOTIVATION JOURNAL

At the end of each of the main chapters is a call to action, and each of these provides some guidance on thoughtful introspection and reflection that you are encouraged to write down for yourself. I recommend that you consider obtaining a journal in which to write your notes and use it as you get to know yourself more fully and begin to apply what you have learned in training your mind to train your body.

Remember, your personal motivation journal is for you; of course, if you feel compelled to share with a friend, that's up to you.

Acknowledgments

Books can be a little less dry with some pictures. So, thanks to my daughter for her good work! Hand-drawn illustrations created by Cassandra Cotter. I would also like to acknowledge my son Matthew Cotter for his assistance in helping me to re-craft and improve the book cover design.

This book presents many stories, experiences and lessons from my life that have contributed to my fitness attitude and my ability to maintain a fitness mindset. I want to take a moment to acknowledge the people who have supported me in this endeavor—namely, my partner Seema who has helped me to maintain my focus and commitment with her belief in my abilities.

I also want to thank my "non-blood" cousin Anastasia, who shared the excitement I felt in making a book like this available for people who struggled staying on the fitness wagon. I also want to thank some of the people who have helped me to understand what it takes to be a trainer, in particular, Mitch Ellis, Michael Sonstein, Mary McNitt and my martial arts co-instructors at Dragon E's Black Belt Academy.

Also, I would like to acknowledge Michelle Vilardi and Kenleigh Paselk and the many other personal trainers who have shared their knowledge and techniques with me as well as supported me in my fitness goals. I am fortunate to have some great medical professionals in my life, and with them in mind, I wish to acknowledge my physician Dr. Adam Buechel DO and also my dentist Dr. Mary Faeth DDS, who have been strong and supportive advocates for me to improve and maintain my health. I would also like to acknowledge and thank my friends and acquaintances who have given me ideas and feedback during the earlier stages of writing this book.

Finally, I would also like to acknowledge my mum Barbara Cotter, my dad Dafydd Cotter for making sure I didn't do too many dangerous things during my childhood so that I could live to tell many tales!

I also give thanks to my sisters Vanessa Burn, Natasha Jackson and Tanya Greenway for being there for me during my first ever running training for the army (and for being such cool sisters) and especially my brother Haydyn Cotter who has always been an inspiration to me with his fierce determination and discipline to exercise and workout, through and in spite of his life-long physical challenges.

I am grateful for all of my family and friends in Australia, and for my extended family and close friends I have gained in America, through my partner, Seema.

Closing thoughts...

You have an awesome opportunity to learn and to re-learn all about yourself.

Use the guidance, write things down in your Personal Motivation Journal and apply what you learn to your fitness journey!

Train the mind to train the body.
Share what you think on Social Media, send me your thoughts, I would be happy to hear from you.

Russell Cotter

Email
author@justmotivateme.org

Website
www.justmotivateme.org

Social media
www.instagram.com/just_motivate_me

www.facebook.com/JMMforfitness

www.linkedin.com/just-motivate-me-for-fitness

My Fitness Protocol

My own protocol that I invented and have used since January 26, 2018:

1. START SLOW. Small, low-intensity exercises. This begins to train your brain to create a mindset where you see exercise can be achievable.

2. CORE IS KING (or QUEEN) If possible, work on your core first and build around it. It makes all the other exercises easier. If you cannot work on your core, moving your body, even gently still counts.

3. MANUFACTURE TIME. No time makes for an easy excuse, so figure out how to get extra time in your day for exercise.

4. MIX IT UP. Don't do the same routine every day. It's boring and you need to work different muscle groups regularly.

5. LEARN FROM AN EXPERT. I have worked with a few great personal trainers, and they were helpful in teaching me new exercises and getting my technique and form right.

6. MATHEMATICS MATTERS. Count your reps, your distances and your time spent, track your progress and celebrate your wins!

7. INTERVAL TRAINING. Regulate your rate of intensity and reps of exercises high and low.

8. GYMS ARE GREAT BUT THEY CAN WAIT. You really don't need an expensive watch or a gym membership. Stairs are free. Floor work is free. Stability balls are cheap.

9. FIND YOUR REASON. Wake-up calls: back pain or a heart attack may induce the motivation you need along with being self-sufficient and not burdening others.

10. MAKE AN ACHIEVABLE SCHEDULE. I do Mondays, Tuesdays, Thursdays and Fridays, walking two to three miles every day when it isn't snowing or raining heavily.

11. KEEP MOVING. Movement keeps blood flowing to the joints, and walking burns calories.

12. STIMULATE YOUR MIND. If you are walking, play a game on your phone (just don't bump into anyone)! If you are working out, play an audiobook.

13. STRETCH AS REST. Just sitting down to get your breath back stops movement and wastes workout time. Use the time for stretches. It's even better when you're already warmed up. Your phone can wait. This is sometimes used as "active recovery"—a little term I picked up from a personal trainer.

Motivational Considerations and Helpers

1. Think about your best time of day to train—mornings, evenings before sleep? What about the time of the week—not on Mondays? Everyone has their own preferences that help with motivation.

2. Accomplish multiple things—household chores can be exercise. Do yard work. Work burns calories and gets stuff done!

3. Vary a normal activity—park your car a little further at the shops or at work. Take the stairs before the elevator when possible.

4. Do exercise that incorporates learning—learning self-defense through martial arts, learning to swim, learning to dance.

5. Find something that is goal oriented and fun—join a scavenger or photo hunt.

6. Take in an inspirational movie or two—*Rocky 1* and *Rocky 2* are among my favorites, but there are many more out there, ones about people running marathons or even comedies about army training like "Stripes" or "Private Benjamin". Oldies but still goodies!

7. Find like-minded people—not fitness junkies, but people who also struggle with motivation—that you can confide in and use mutual accountability to make a good go of training together!

8. Set a goal but not *just for* fitness—huh? What I mean is to set a goal that will *demand* a level of fitness. It might be to take a hike or to qualify for a better life insurance premium. A goal might also be to have the energy to play with kids or grandkids!

9. Take your next streaming video binge watch *with* you—if you have a smartphone or tablet, then maybe do your binge watching while stepping on the treadmill or working out on an elliptical machine.

10. Create your affirmation and wear it—a word on a pendant, maybe even a tattoo or a t-shirt.

Also, remember: The website www.justmotivateme.org is something that complements the book and also is my way of helping folks through their journey, the one we all share. You will find blog posts, mini mindful motivation videos, merchandise and games and insights.